Contents

About the authors   **v**

Acknowledgements   **vi**

Introduction   **1**
    Overall aim of the programme   1
    Objectives of this book   1
    Self-assessment of where you are now with clinical
        effectiveness and clinical governance   2
    What are clinical effectiveness and evidence-based
        healthcare?   5
    What is the evidence for evidence-based healthcare?   6
    Why health professionals need information   7
    Are clinicians ready for evidence-based healthcare?   8
    Learning by portfolio   9
    Electronic databases   11

Stage 1: Asking the right question   **19**
    Questions about cost-effectiveness   20
    Framing questions: some examples   22

Stage 2: Undertaking a literature search   **28**
    The search strategy: think, search and appraise   28
    Undertake a search   29
    Using the Cochrane Library   30
    Using the Medline database   31
    The hierarchy of evidence   32
    Examples   33
    Searching by yourself   42

Stage 3: Frame your own question and search for the evidence   **47**

Stage 4: Appraise the evidence   **51**
    The meaning of different research methods and terms   51
    Reading a paper   58
    Critical appraisal of a published paper or report of a study   59
    Examples   62
    Critical appraisal of a qualitative research paper   73
    Critically appraise a review   75
    Our review of *Br J Gen Pract* 1997; **47**: 647–52   77

Stage 5: Apply the evidence   **82**
    Diary of your progress in searching for evidence   82
    Action plan   83
    Barriers to change   84

**Stage 6: What clinical governance means and how to put it
into practice**   **86**
    Components of clinical governance   86
    The challenges to delivering clinical governance   88
    Enhancing your personal and professional development   89
    How evidence-based care, clinical effectiveness and other
    components of clinical governance fit together:
    • the practitioner's, the practice's or the unit's perspective   91
    • the primary care organisation's or trust's perspective   102
    • Research Governance Framework for Health and Social Care   108

**Evaluate your newly gained knowledge and skills in clinical
effectiveness and clinical governance**   **112**

Useful publications of evidence already available   **115**
    Organisations   116
    Further reading   117

References   **119**

Index   **123**

CLINICAL EFFECTIVENESS
AND CLINICAL GOVERNANCE
MADE EASY

Fourth Edition

Ruth Chambers

Elizabeth Boath

and David Rogers

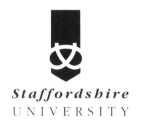

Staffordshire
UNIVERSITY

RADCLIFFE PUBLISHING

Radcliffe Publishing Ltd
18 Marcham Road
Abingdon
Oxon OX14 1AA
United Kingdom

www.radcliffe-oxford.com
Electronic catalogue and worldwide online ordering facility.

First edition 1998
Second edition 2001
Third edition 2004

British Library Cataloguing in Publication Data

A catalogue record for this book is available from the British Library.

ISBN-13: 978 1 84619 146 6

Typeset by Advance Typesetting Ltd, Oxford
Printed and bound by TJI Digital, Padstow, Cornwall

About the authors

Ruth Chambers has been a general practitioner for more than 20 years. She is currently Director of GP Education at West Midlands Workforce Deanery and Professor of Primary Care Development at Staffordshire University. Her interest in clinical effectiveness and clinical audit grew from her three-year spell as Chairman of Staffordshire Medical Audit Advisory Group in the 1990s.

Ruth has run several series of clinical effectiveness and clinical governance workshops, teaching a mix of primary and community care health professionals clinical effectiveness skills in easy steps and an understanding of clinical governance. The experiences of those workshops have informed this book.

Elizabeth Boath is Reader in Health at the Faculty of Health, Staffordshire University. Her interest in clinical effectiveness grew from her time as a primary and community care research facilitator, during which she facilitated and taught on the series of clinical effectiveness workshops used to develop this book.

David Rogers is the clinical effectiveness librarian for the Bedside Clinical Guidelines Partnership. He has taught thousands of health professionals how to seek for the evidence base for their practice over the years. David also provides the evidence for clinical guidelines used by 15 hospital trusts across the Midlands and beyond.

Acknowledgements

The book was originally based on the experiences from running two series of four workshops, *Clinical Effectiveness Made Easy*, for primary and community care practitioners and 20 workshops about *Clinical Governance*. We are grateful to the participants of the workshops for contributing so many ideas and being such enthusiastic health professionals. Irene Fenton, local lead healthcare librarian, provided the inspiration and clear advice about undertaking literature searches and other sources of evidence.

We are grateful to Nicky Macleod for her contribution about the meaning of cost-effectiveness, and Dr Gill Wakley, who helped to devise and facilitate the clinical governance workshops.

Ruth Chambers
Elizabeth Boath
David Rogers
February 2007

Introduction

Clinical effectiveness and clinical governance are about knowing what you should be doing and being able to put that knowledge into practice

Overall aim of the programme

To increase awareness of, and skills in, the adoption of an evidence-based approach to the practice and delivery of healthcare.

Objectives of this book

This programme is for all health professionals to learn how to:

- ask the right question – it must be important to you and your colleagues
- look for the evidence and do a literature search
- receive and incorporate constructive criticism from colleagues about their developing questions and search for evidence
- select the best evidence – what to do where no strong evidence exists
- evaluate and interpret the evidence, such as read and extract information from a report
- apply the evidence as appropriate in a practice, unit or department
- act on the evidence to improve the practice of clinical effectiveness
- promote a culture of clinical governance.

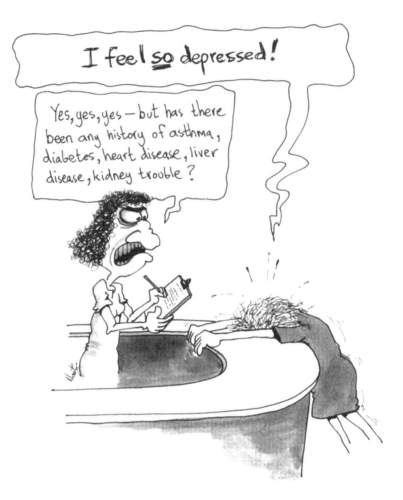

Do you need to update your style of practice?

Self-assessment of where you are now with clinical effectiveness and clinical governance

Before you start working through the clinical effectiveness and clinical governance programme, assess your baseline knowledge and attitudes. You should complete a similar self-assessment when you have worked through the book, so that you can compare your answers to see how your knowledge and skills have increased. Please circle as many answers as apply, or fill in the information requested.

1 How confident do you feel that you are capable of practising clinical effectiveness to be able to:

ask a relevant question?	*Very*	*Somewhat*	*Not at all*
undertake a search of the literature?	*Very*	*Somewhat*	*Not at all*
find readily available evidence?	*Very*	*Somewhat*	*Not at all*
weigh up available evidence?	*Very*	*Somewhat*	*Not at all*
decide if changes in practice are warranted?	*Very*	*Somewhat*	*Not at all*
make changes in practice as appropriate?	*Very*	*Somewhat*	*Not at all*

2 Have you ever searched the literature yourself for an answer to a question?   *Yes/No*

If '*Yes*':

• which database(s) have you used?

Medline   Cochrane   OMNI   Other (what?)

• where did you search the literature?

Medical library   At work   At home   Other (where?)

• did you have any help in searching the literature?

None   Healthcare librarian   Friend/family   Work colleague   Other (who?)

3 Have you ever asked someone else to search the literature for you? *Yes/No*

If '*Yes*':

• who did the search for you?
• why didn't you do the search yourself?

*Lack of time   Lack of skill   Lack of access   Other reason
to databases*

4 Can you complete the following list from your own knowledge, describing the features of different types or levels of evidence in decreasing order of robustness from very strong evidence to none at all?

Type	Features
I	Strong evidence from at least one systematic review of multiple, well-designed, randomised controlled trials
II	
III	
IV	
V	Opinions of respected authorities, descriptive studies, reports of experts

5 If you have previously searched for the evidence to answer a question you had posed, what did you do with the result of your search? (Circle all that apply.)

- *Discussed it with colleagues at work*
- *Discussed it with friends or family*
- *Made change(s) to an aspect of work*
- *Decided against making any change(s) to any aspect of work*
- *Other outcome – what?*

6 To what extent is evidence-based healthcare central to your own practice? (Circle all that apply.)

- *I have no idea whether my everyday practice is evidence-based most of the time*
- *I assume that my everyday practice is evidence-based whenever possible, but I've no evidence for that assumption*
- *I ensure that my everyday practice is evidence-based by regularly comparing my practice against published standards of best practice and making appropriate changes*

7 How many of these principles of good practice in clinical governance do you generally include as part of your quality improvement work? (Circle all that apply.)

- *I actively promote or participate in multidisciplinary working*
- *I address national, local, organisational or professional priorities in my work*
- *I try to achieve partnership working, e.g. between agencies, between management/clinicians*
- *I incorporate input from patients in my work (e.g. users, carers, the public) in training, planning, monitoring or delivery of healthcare*
- *I look for potential to achieve health gains in the way I organise my work*
- *My everyday work is based on evidence-based practice, policy or management*
- *I can demonstrate the standards of care or services that I or my team achieve*

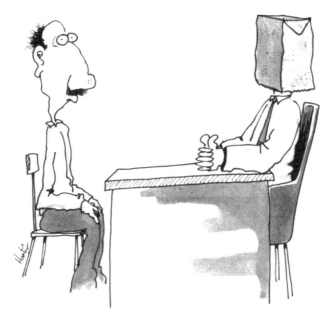

**Find out how to practise clinical effectiveness – don't shut your eyes
to the changes going on around you.**

What are clinical effectiveness and evidence-based healthcare?

Clinical effectiveness is 'the extent to which specific clinical interventions, when deployed in the field for a particular patient or population, do what they are intended to do – i.e. maintain and improve health and secure the greatest possible health gain from the available resources. To be reasonably certain that an intervention has produced health benefits, it needs to be shown to be capable of producing worthwhile benefit (efficacy and cost-effectiveness) and that it has produced that benefit in practice'.[1]

Evidence-based healthcare 'takes place when decisions that affect the care of patients are taken with due weight accorded to all valid, relevant information'.[2]

Evidence-based healthcare is the 'conscientious, explicit, and judicious use of current best evidence in making decisions about the care of individual patients. The practice of evidence-based medicine means integrating individual clinical expertise with the best available external clinical evidence from systematic research'.[3]

A problem-solving approach based on good evidence can also be applied to non-clinical decision making, such as most areas of management and resource allocation, as well as to clinical situations.

The three components of best possible clinical decision making[4,5] are *clinical expertise, patient preferences* and *clinical research evidence*. Clinical expertise and patient preferences may override the research evidence in some situations and for some patients. For example, patients may opt for less invasive treatment, or a sick patient may be too frail to undergo treatment with significant side effects.

Clinical audit remains an important tool for determining whether actual performance compares with evidence-based standards and, if not, what changes are needed to improve performance. Clinical audit is 'the systematic and critical analysis of the quality of clinical care, including the procedures used for diagnosis, treatment and care, the associated use of resources and the resulting outcome and quality of life for the patient'.[1] In other words, clinical audit helps you to reach a standard of clinical work as near to best practice as possible.

The process of achieving evidence-based healthcare can be divided into four sections:

1 the composition of a good question
2 a search of the literature to find the 'best' evidence available
3 an evaluation of what seems to be the most appropriate and relevant literature
4 the application of the evidence or findings.

What is the evidence for evidence-based healthcare?

There is growing evidence for the implementation of evidence-based health-care.[6] Promoting Action on Clinical Effectiveness (PACE), a King's Fund programme, developed evidence-based practice as a routine way of working for health services. An interim report[6] described the successful outcomes when clinical effectiveness was linked to local needs and priorities so long as clinicians, managers, policy makers and patients were all involved in the process.

Practising in an evidence-based way:

- will promote your job satisfaction and feeling of being in control over your work
- can be used to justify maintaining or increasing budget allocations to particular areas of work
- will enhance your capability to do what's best for the patient.[7]

Why health professionals need information

Health professionals need to be well informed to be able to advise and inform patients appropriately. Patients who access the Internet and other electronic databases are starting to use that information to challenge clinicians' decisions about their care.

Clinicians will come under more pressure to respond to patients who have easy access to detailed information obtained from various sources, some of which will be inaccurate and misleading. The movement to patient empowerment has been generally welcomed, but may be threatening for clinicians who are insufficiently prepared to talk to well-informed patients, because they are unsure of their own knowledge base, time pressured, or do not understand how to assess what is the best evidence.

Clinicians will need to develop skills in finding and judging medical information, and communicating such information to patients appropriately. Health professionals may lay themselves open to complaints or legal procedures if they fail to adopt best practice through ignorance of the available evidence. Clinicians need good communication skills as well as reliable information when advising patients.

Patients are increasingly encouraged to seek out information from the Internet themselves. Health professionals can help patients by indicating which electronic sources are most likely to be appropriate and reliable.

Ultimately, reliable and accurate information, good communication skills and patient empowerment are all features of a good quality primary healthcare service and a positive culture of clinical governance. Health professionals and managers need good information when assessing the health needs of their patient populations, commissioning healthcare services and striving to reduce inequalities. Detailed information is needed to distinguish between different subgroups of the population, between patient populations and others elsewhere, or to monitor variations in performance between different practitioners and general practices or hospitals.

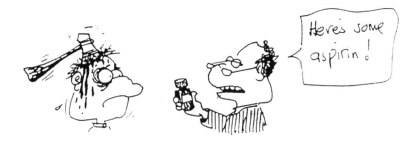

Quality of care may be compromised ...

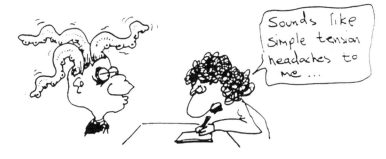

without clinical effectiveness

Are clinicians ready for evidence-based healthcare?

Surveys of general practitioners' perceptions of evidence-based healthcare in the late 1990s[7,8] found that GPs knew little about extracting information from journals, review publications and databases, and that few who were knowledgeable used these sources of information. The majority of GPs welcomed evidence-based healthcare and agreed that it improves patient care.[7] GPs have been found to be more aware of publications that summarise evidence,[9] such as *Bandolier* rather than electronic databases. The researchers[7] concluded that the way forward in encouraging primary care clinicians to adopt evidence-based healthcare lay in promoting and improving access to summaries of evidence, and encouraging those primary care clinicians who are skilled in accessing and interpreting evidence to develop local evidence-based guidelines and advice.

One study[8] concluded that what was needed was a culture whereby health professionals posed 'regular questions about the validity of patient care' and developed 'skills both in defining useful questions and finding the answers'.

When GPs were asked what training they wanted in evidence-based practice, just over half wanted training in the use of databases.[8]

Adverse comments about evidence-based practice include fear of the imposition of too rigid a healthcare culture, the loss of an overriding duty to provide compassionate and sensitive care[10] and that wholesale evidence-based practice is unrealistic because it is not affordable. Some people mistrust the research–evidence base component of evidence-based practice because of the unreliability of some of the published literature; study biases are not always sufficiently recognised or acknowledged and, in occasional cases, have been discredited by sensational scandals involving researchers falsifying data.

Putting evidence into practice is a long and complicated process. Research from the King's Fund and others has emphasised that success in applying evidence-based practice is more likely: if there are sufficient resources (time, money and skills); if the proposed changes offer benefits to frontline staff; if the right people are 'signed up' to the proposed changes early enough; if the change is managed in an interactive way; and if research underpinning the change is clearly related to practice.[11,12] Many different approaches are being tried to overcome practitioners' and managers' seeming reluctance to change their practice according to new evidence as research is published. Governments are translating their policies into practical guidance and toolkits for implementing national standards or frameworks.[13,14] But we have a long way to go before the policies that governments evolve are evidence-based themselves.[15]

Learning by portfolio

Portfolio-based learning has been promoted since the early 1990s as a style of education that allows individuals to progress at their own pace. People can adopt education relevant to their needs, and composing a portfolio allows plenty of opportunities for reflection. Portfolio-based learning is not an easy option[16] compared to relatively passive types of learning such as listening to lectures. It takes a great deal of effort to complete a successful portfolio built on your past experiences and to progress through the stages of gathering and processing new information, critical reflection, interpretation and application. But it is worth it. The satisfaction that comes from completing a portfolio is as much about being in control of your own education as acquiring new knowledge, attitudes and/or skills.[17,18]

Another advantage of composing a portfolio is that on-the-job learning is relevant to your work and life, and this is likely to retain your interest. At the end of the project you will have discovered that you have further educational and developmental needs. And hopefully you will be discussing these within your annual appraisal. You will then have to decide whether or not you have taken learning about this topic, i.e. how to practise clinical effectiveness, as far as your resources (time, cost and effort) permit.

So, using a portfolio-based approach to acquire the basic ability to practise clinical effectiveness, you should aim in your work programme to:

- identify the learning task(s), e.g. what capability you need to be able to practise clinical effectiveness and clinical governance
- set learning goals, e.g. learn to frame a question; search for, interpret and apply the evidence
- identify ways of achieving your goals by, for example, working through this book, peer group discussion, visiting colleagues, undertaking a (supervised) literature search, exploring the Internet, reading more widely, making changes at work. Use this information to compose your personal development plan
- identify learning resources, e.g. electronic databases in the healthcare library, the Internet, books, journals, video tuition tapes, local courses, correspondence from hospital specialists
- monitor how well the learning is going, e.g. reflect on the development of your knowledge and skills, seek a colleague's view of your work. Work with others in your practice or at the trust to feed your learning needs into the workplace development plan
- list your achievements, e.g. run through a cycle of clinical effectiveness
- use what you have learned, e.g. make change(s) at work as a result of obtaining evidence or new information as part of clinical governance.

Some people prefer to work alone, while others find that having a mentor to help build the portfolio is useful. A mentor can help you to determine your learning needs, develop a study plan, support and challenge the work done, identify further learning gaps and generally help you to stay on course. To some extent the way that this clinical effectiveness learning programme is set out obviates the need for a mentor, but if you think a mentor might facilitate your work, consider asking your line manager or local tutor to recommend a mentor; or maybe a colleague could work alongside you sharing the 'programme' too, as a 'co-mentor' or 'buddy'.[16]

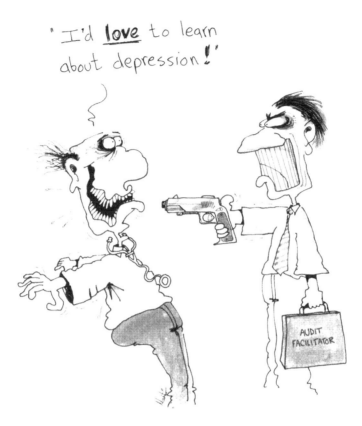

Clinical effectiveness requires real commitment.

Electronic databases

The Internet

The Internet is the largest computer network in the world to which almost any type of computer can link. Most academic institutions are connected to the Joint Academic Network (JANET) and its Internet service (JIPS); staff and students can then access the Internet free on campus, or can dial up from home via a modem for the cost of a local phone call. NHSNet is the equivalent for all NHSstaff.

Information can be extracted from the Internet or exchanged via the World Wide Web (www) by electronic mail, newsgroups and file transfer protocol (ftp). The World Wide Web is a system for providing access to a network of interlinked documents and information services across the Internet. Documents can be stored on the Web as text, images, sound or video. The language that the Web clients and servers use to communicate with each other is called 'hypertext transfer protocol' (http).

To use the World Wide Web you need software called a *browser* (or *client*) to view www documents, such as Navigator or Microsoft Internet Explorer. The latter is included with Windows, and the latest versions of both can be freely downloaded from the Web. If you want to read more about what informatics can do for you, read *The Clinician's Guide to Surviving IT*.[19]

There is now a large number of Internet Service Providers (ISPs), with the early ISPs such as AOL and CompuServe having been joined by others like BTInternet and TescoNet. The wide availability of broadband access has made using the Internet much more efficient and is rapidly superseding 'dial up'.

Medline

Medline is produced by the National Library of Medicine in the United States and is freely available to all (without a password) via the PubMed website: www.ncbi.nlm.nih.gov/entrez/query.fcgi?DB=pubmed

Other ways of searching Medline on the Web include the Dialog interface for all NHS staff * (ask your health library for a password or use the Athens self-registration function), or the Ebsco interface for university students or staff.

Medline contains over 12 million citations dating from 1950 to the present, from more than 4600 biomedical journals published in the United States and 70 other countries. Author abstracts are available for about 80% of the entries. It covers the whole field of medicine, dentistry, veterinary medicine, medical psychology, nursing, the healthcare system, and the pre-clinical sciences. Coverage is worldwide, but most records are from English-language sources or have English abstracts.

Cochrane Library

The Cochrane Library (www.nelh.nhs.uk/cochrane.asp) is considered to be the single best source of reliable evidence about the effects of healthcare.[20] The Cochrane Library includes:

- The Cochrane Database of Systematic Reviews (CDSR). These are structured, systematic reviews of controlled trials. Evidence is included or

---

* http://nhs.dialog.com/

excluded according to explicit quality criteria. A meta-analysis is undertaken by combining data from different studies to increase the *power* of the findings.

- The Database of Abstracts of Reviews of Effects (DARE). This is a database of research reviews of the effectiveness of healthcare interventions and the management and organisation of health services. The reviews are critically appraised by reviewers at the NHS Centre for Reviews and Dissemination at the University of York.
- The Cochrane Central Register of Controlled Trials (CENTRAL). This bibliography of controlled trials has been compiled by both database and hand searches through the world's literature. The Register includes reports from conference proceedings.

This original core of the Cochrane Library has now been supplemented by the addition of: the NHS Economic Evaluation Database (NHSEED), Health Technology Assessment Database (HTA) and Cochrane Methodology Register (CMR). The Cochrane Library was freely available to all via the National Library for Health (NLH) at: www.nelh.nhs.uk/cochrane.asp, but following the adoption of a new interface hosted by the publishers Wiley, access is currently restricted to the Database of Systematic Reviews only. Negotiations to restore full access are currently underway.

EMBASE

The Excerpta Medica database (EMBASE) is the largest competitor to Medline, but has a European bias in contrast to its rival's US bias. It contains over 7.5 million documents from 1974 to the present, indexed from over 4000 journals, and over 80% of entries have author abstracts. The overlap of coverage with Medline is around 40%, so a search on EMBASE will often recover papers not found on Medline. EMBASE has a similar subject coverage to Medline, but is stronger on pharmacology and therapeutics. Unlike Medline, which enjoys state subsidisation, EMBASE is produced commercially by the Dutch company Elsevier, and has consequently been too expensive in the past for all but the biggest of libraries to provide. However, EMBASE is now available as part of the NHSCore Content via Dialog (see your health library for a password).

CINAHL

The Cumulative Index to Nursing and Allied Health Literature (CINAHL) database, compiled by CINAHL Information Systems in the USA, is a comprehensive database of more than 1200 English language journals from 1982 to the present. Some foreign language material has been included since 1994. CINAHL covers all aspects of nursing and allied health disciplines, such as health education, occupational therapy, physical therapy, emergency services, and social services and healthcare. Selected journals are also indexed in the areas of consumer health, biomedicine and health sciences librarianship. The database also provides access to healthcare books, nursing dissertations, selected conference proceedings, standards of professional practice, educational software and audio-visual materials in nursing. CINAHL has more than 7000 records with full text and 1200 records with images. Approximately 70% of CINAHL headings also appear in Medline. CINAHL supplements these headings with 4000+ terms designed specifically for nursing and allied health disciplines. For more information, see the following website: www.cinahl.com

Several studies have compared Medline and CINAHL. These revealed that while Medline assigns more index terms to each article, CINAHL uses index terms that are more focused on nursing and therapy topics.[21] Another study revealed that CINAHL was preferred by nursing students as it gave a higher number of relevant articles, while a further study found that both databases were relevant for allied health professionals (AHPs).[22,23] The authors concluded that, in order to ensure a comprehensive search, both Medline and CINAHL should be used. CINAHL is available via Dialog (see your health library for a password).

Subject-specific bibliographic databases[24,25]

Over 2 000 000 articles are published each year in over 20 000 medical and related journals. Thus, although electronic databases provide access to references from a large number of journals, no database provides access to all journals. So, if you search only one or two databases, you might miss a relevant article. In addition to searching the main databases, it is also worthwhile searching any specialist databases relevant to your area of interest. Some of these databases are outlined in alphabetical order below.

- **AgeLine** covers ageing, middle age and the elderly, and includes research on psychology, public policy, healthcare, business, gerontology and consumer issues. The information has a US bias but it is possible to limit to a particular target audience, e.g. patients or professionals. AgeLine is freely available at: http://research.aarp.org/ageline
- The databases formerly known as **AIDSDRUGS**, **AIDSTRIALS** and **AIDSLINE** are now searchable as a subset of PubMed via the NLM gateway at: http://gateway.nlm.nih.gov
- **AMED** (Allied and Alternative Medicine), available as part of the NHSCore Content via Dialog (see your health library for a password), searches across

the spectrum of complementary and alternative medicine. It covers articles from 400 journals, many of which are not indexed elsewhere, from 1985 to the present.

- **ASSIA plus** (Applied Social Sciences Index and Abstracts) covers all major social sciences and related media, including sociology, social policy, psychology and relevant aspects of anthropology, economics, medicine, law and politics. It features over 312 000 records from over 650 English language journals, covering 16 countries, including 25 of the 30 most cited sources. It covers the period since 1987 and is updated monthly. It is available (on subscription only) from Cambridge Scientific Abstracts Internet Database Service. See www.csa.com/factsheets/assia-set-c.php for more details.

- **CANCERLIT** – the database formerly known as CANCERLIT is now available as a subset of PubMed at www.cancer.gov/search/cancer_literature

- **Clinical Evidence** is a compendium of the best available evidence on the effects of common clinical interventions and is freely available to all via the National Library for Health (NLH) at: www.clinicalevidence.com/ceweb/conditions/index.jsp

- **EDINA BIOSIS** covers more than 6500 journals from more than 90 countries from 1985 to the present. It covers biological sciences and related subjects, including public health. It is updated every week and over 500 000 articles are added annually. EDINA offers the UK tertiary education and research community networked access to a library of data, information and research resources. All EDINA services were available free of charge to members of UK tertiary education institutions for academic use. Institutional subscription and personal registration is required. Go to the ISI Web of Knowledge Service for UK Education at: http://wos.mimas.ac.uk/

- **PsycINFO**® includes worldwide literature from 1887 to the present in the field of psychology and psychological aspects of related disciplines, including medicine, psychiatry, nursing, sociology, education, pharmacology, physiology, linguistics, anthropology, business and law. PsycINFO is updated monthly and covers 1300 journals in 25 languages – over 45 000 references are added annually. PsycINFO is available as part of the NHS Core Content via Dialog (see your health library for a password).

- **SUMSearch** is a unique method for searching the Internet for EBM information. It queries a variety of databases including Medline, the National Guideline Clearinghouse from the Agency for Health Care Policy and Research (AHCPR) and DARE. SUMSearch automatically corrects common abbreviations and common terms that are hard to search for on common databases. For example, it converts *DVT* to *deep vein thrombosis* and *heart failure* to *heart failure or ventricular failure* – small changes that

greatly affect Medline search results. It is freely available at: http://
sumsearch.uthscsa.edu

Other information on the Internet[24,25]

- **Bath Information and Data Service (BIDS)**[19] at www.bids.ac.uk is a
  database designed to be used by non-expert searchers and includes several
  medically orientated databases such as EMBASE, Citation Indexes and Inside
  Information, with a wide variety of medically related reference material.
  BIDS is at present only available to staff and students in the higher
  education community. As well as providing database access free at the
  point of delivery, a large number of full-text electronic journals, with links
  to database search results in many cases, are also available.
- **Health on the Net** at www.hon.ch The Health on the Net Foundation, a
  Swiss non-governmental organisation, has developed a code of conduct
  (HON code) for medical and health websites. This states that medical
  information should either be given by medically trained and qualified
  professionals or, if this is not possible, it should be indicated clearly that the
  information is given by non-medically qualified people. Websites com-
  plying with this code bear the Health on the Net logo. But the presence of a
  logo is not a guarantee of the quality of the information. A meta-search
  engine (one that searches many databases simultaneously) called
  MedHunt is supplied on the homepage.
- **Medical Matrix** at www.medmatrix.org This database is available only
  on subscription, lists over 6000 quality-assessed medical websites and links
  to over 1.5 million documents.
- The **National Research Register** (NRR) is a register of ongoing or
  recently completed research and development projects funded by, or of
  interest to, the NHS. It also contains details of reviews in progress collected
  by the NHS Centre for Reviews and Dissemination (CRD). The current
  release (Issue 2 of 2006) contains information on 151 120 research
  projects, as well as entries from the Medical Research Council's Clinical
  Trials Directory. The NRR is assembled and published by Update Software
  Ltd on behalf of the Department of Health in the United Kingdom. The
  complete NRR database is free on the Internet at www.nrr.nhs.uk/
  search.htm
- **ReFeR**, the Department of Health Research Findings Register, helps to fill
  the gap between research completion and publication by providing details
  of the findings of many projects listed in the National Research Register. It is
  freely available via the NLH at: www.refer.nhs.uk/
- **PubMed** is the National Library of Medicine's search service that was
  developed in conjunction with publishers of biomedical literature as a

search tool for accessing literature citations and linking to full-text journals at websites of participating publishers. It provides access to over 12 000 000 citations in Medline, PreMedline (updated daily, providing basic citation information and abstracts before the citation is indexed and added to Medline), NLM Gateway and other related databases, with links to participating online journals and textbooks. The NLM Gateway also gives access to OldMedline, which indexes journal articles from 1950 to 1965. Although searching PubMed is free, user registration, a subscription fee, or fee at the point of use may be required to access the full text of articles in some journals. It is available at www.ncbi.nlm.nih.gov/entrez/query.fcgi?DB= pubmed

• The **TRIP+** database is a one-stop search engine for evidence-based material on the Internet and is available only on subscription, although your higher education institution may have Athens access. www.update-software.com/scripts/clibng/html/tripusernamelogon.htm

Website for learning evidence-based healthcare skills[26]

The Centre for Evidence Based Medicine at Oxford includes a useful 'toolbox' and also downloads of free materials on its website at www.cebm.net/

Useful software

Mentor Plus[27] is an electronic medical knowledge clinical support system originally developed by Oxford University Press with EMIS (Egton Medical Information Systems Ltd). It has information about more than 2000 diseases cross-referenced with about 26 000 commonly used medical terms. The programme comes up with a differential diagnosis for a set of symptoms, signs and test results, suggesting appropriate management plans which are a mix of evidence-based medicine and best practice. EMIS is now offering an updated version, 'Web Mentor Libary' as a subscription service costing at present £74 plus VAT per annum.

Electronic journals

The situation regarding access to the full text of online journals is complicated and ever-changing. Ask your healthcare librarian for details. Some of the websites show the full contents of the journal, others do not carry the full text of all original articles.

- *British Medical Journal* www.bmj.com (is now freely available for the current issue only, although your institution may have Athens access to full text).

As part of the NHS Core Content package, Proquest and some other agents provide access to over 1200 full-text journals with links to Dialog database search results. Ask your health library for an Athens password to use this service.

Higher education users will have access to a different package of electronic journals, usually needing an Athens password. Your university or college library can provide details.

'The greatest obstacle to discovering the truth is being convinced that you already know it.'

Stage 1

Asking the right question[28]

Although you may be burning to ask your question, when you actually try to set it down on paper, you may find that the exercise is more difficult than you think.

Questions have to be phrased in a very specific way to obtain meaningful responses in any context. This applies to asking other people what they think about a topic as much as for searching the literature for the best evidence.

The best clinical questions relate to queries arising from your own patients during the course of your work rather than being hypothetical questions. Relevant work-based questions should motivate you to seek the evidence and make change(s). Before you go to a lot of trouble to find answers or solutions to your questions, ask around at work and find out if anyone else is concerned about the same question or problem, already has the answer(s), or knows where to find them.

The question should be:

- simple
- specific
- realistic
- important
- capable of being answered
- agreed and owned by those who will be involved in any changes resulting
- implementable
- about a topic where change will be possible.

Think about how to construct your clinical question by considering:

- what the question is about. For example, is the question about an individual or group of patients? What are the patient characteristics you are interested in, such as age or gender? Is it a clinical dilemma or a resource problem?
- the setting. For example, is it specific to primary, secondary or community care, rural or urban locations?
- the type of intervention and whether it is being compared with current practice or another intervention. For example, are you interested in different treatments, causes, prognostic factors or risks, compared with current practice or no treatment?

- the outcome(s) of the clinical topic. For example, is an acceptable outcome to your question reduced numbers of cases of diseases, reduced patients' suffering, or increased quality of life?

You should focus and phrase your question to include whatever it is that you want to know about effects, efficiency, diagnosis or prognosis. You may decide to have a main question with several subsidiary questions.

Questions about cost-effectiveness

Cost-effectiveness is not synonymous with 'cheap'. A cost-effective intervention is one which gives a better or equivalent benefit from the intervention in question for lower or equivalent cost, or where the relative improvement in outcome is higher than the relative difference in cost. In other words, being cost-effective means having the best outcomes for the least input. Using the term 'cost-effective' implies that you have considered potential alternatives.

An intervention must first be considered *clinically* effective to warrant investigation into its potential to be *cost*-effective. Evidence-based practice must incorporate clinical judgement. You have to interpret the evidence when it comes to applying it to individual patients, whether it be evidence about clinical effectiveness or cost-effectiveness.

If you want to ask a question about cost-effectiveness you should be sure to have confirmed clinical effectiveness first, and have gone on to ask a question about cost-effectiveness as the second stage in seeking the evidence.

A 'benefit' is what is gained from meeting a chosen need and a 'cost' is the benefit that would have been obtained from using the same resources in an alternative way. Opportunity costs are the costs of the benefits foregone in deploying resources in the chosen way. They are the value of the benefits given up in the next best use of those resources.[29]

A new or alternative treatment or intervention should be compared directly with the next best treatment or intervention.

An economic evaluation is a comparative analysis of two or more alternatives in terms of their costs and consequences.[29,30] There are four different types: cost-effectiveness, cost minimisation, cost–utility analysis and cost–benefit analysis. Cost-effectiveness analysis is used to compare the effectiveness of two interventions with the same treatment objectives. Cost minimisation compares the costs of alternative treatments which have identical health outcomes. Cost–utility analysis enables the effects of alternative interventions to be measured against a combination of life expectancy and quality of life, a common outcome measure being 'quality-adjusted life-years' (QALYs). A cost–benefit analysis compares the incremental costs and benefits of a programme.

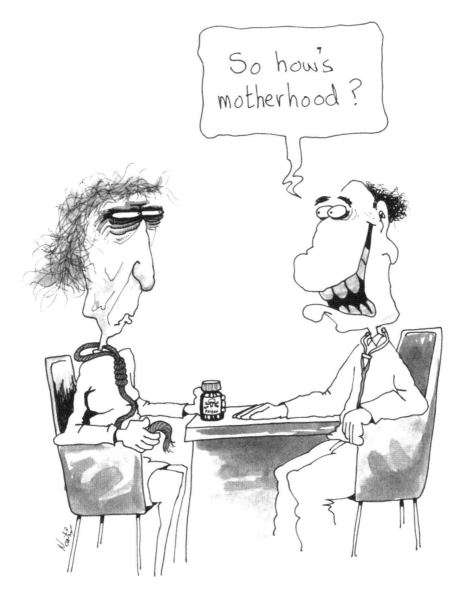

Asking inappropriate questions.

Efficiency is sometimes confused with effectiveness. Being efficient means having obtained the most quality from the least expenditure, or the required level of quality for the least expenditure. To measure efficiency you need to make a judgement about the level of quality of the 'purchase' and be able to relate it to 'price'. 'Price' alone does not measure efficiency. Quality is the indicator used in combination with price to assess whether something is more efficient.

So, cost-effectiveness is a measure of efficiency and suggests that costs have been related to effectiveness.

> 'I have finally made up my mind but the decision was by no means unanimous.'

Framing questions: some examples

Now try these two examples of clinical situations and frame a specific question for each with which you might search the literature for evidence to answer the question.

Jot down notes under each heading and write the final question at the bottom of the page ready to do a trial literature search using the Medline database. Refine and limit the question to what would seem to be a relevant question for those working in primary care. Your question should be shaped by thinking about exactly why you are asking it and how you might apply the evidence in practice once you have obtained it.

Set a question to address problem 1

A general practice is taking stock of the preventive work it does and is reviewing whether to continue the range of work that different health professionals offer. The staff are wondering what impact the range of health education about smoking that they offer has on their patients.

1 What is the question about – an individual patient, a group of people, a particular population, patient characteristics, a clinical dilemma, a re-source problem?

2 What is the setting or context of the clinical topic/situation?

3 Is there an intervention and, if so, with what is it being compared?

4 What is/are the desired outcome(s) of the clinical intervention?

5 What is the specific question you will ask?

6 Choose up to five key words, in priority order, that you think best represent the important components of your question and restrict them as far as possible to your field of enquiry.

Some example details follow.

Example details of question posed to address problem 1

Defining the question

The refined question should narrow down the limits of the enquiry by specifying as many of the following details as apply:

- What is the question about – the whole or a section of the practice population? What is meant by health education? Which staff are involved with the health education intervention? What is meant by 'smoking' (it could be tobacco or cannabis, cigarettes or cigars, etc.)?
- What is the setting or context of the enquiry? The focus of your interest might be general practice, the community or primary care; or a particular type of clinic in the practice.
- Is there an intervention and, if so, with what is it being compared? What types of health education is the questioner interested in? Is there an alternative model to which health education is being compared?
- What is/are the outcome(s) of the health education intervention and what is meant by 'impact' (e.g. changes in attitudes, knowledge of the adverse effects of smoking, or quantity of cigarettes smoked; reduction in disease severity or frequency)?
- The specific question will have narrowed down the problem to one in which the practice staff are interested. For instance, if the staff in the practice were reviewing whether to continue the teenage lifestyles clinic, besides looking at attendance figures, patient preferences and opportunity costs for staff, the practice team might want to know 'what is the evidence for the

effectiveness of giving adolescents face-to-face education about the risks of cigarette smoking in nurse-run clinics?' A more general question might be 'what is the evidence for the effectiveness of a health professional advising a smoker to stop smoking?'

- Key words might be *health education, smoking, primary healthcare, adolescents*, etc. depending on your question. You might have other key words.

Comments from participants' experiences at the live workshops on clinical effectiveness

Participants found that each small group composed entirely different questions as they had different foci of interests. Some found that their final question did not contain the key words they selected when framing their question, as they had not refined their ideas sufficiently. The result was that in some cases a later search on the chosen key words on Medline missed the point of the question.

Set a question to address problem 2

A mother asks a health professional about her child's eczema and whether it is worth going to all the bother of trying to minimise the amount of house dust lying around at home.

Have a go at completing parts of the question for problem 2:

1 What is the question about – an individual patient, a group of people, a particular population, patient characteristics, a clinical dilemma, a resource problem?

2 What is the setting or context of the clinical topic/situation?

3 Is there an intervention and, if so, with what is it being compared?

4 What is/are the desired outcome(s) of the clinical intervention?

5 What is the specific question you will ask?

6 Choose up to five key words, in priority order, that you think best represent the important components of your question and restrict them as far as possible to your field of enquiry.

Some example details follow.

Example details of question posed to address problem 2

Defining the question

A refined question will narrow down the limits of the enquiry by specifying as many of the following details as apply:

- What is the question about – the child or the practice population as a whole? What is meant by house dust – or house dust mite? What is meant by eczema? Is there any other condition that it would be important to search on, e.g. asthma?
- What is the setting or context of the enquiry? The focus of your interest might be general practice, the community or primary care.
- If there is an intervention, with what is it being compared – the method of eradication of house dust, or any other type of intervention such as other treatments for eczema?
- What is/are the outcome(s) of the health education intervention and what is meant by *minimise* – changes in symptoms, reduction in frequency of flare-ups, etc.?
- The specific question should narrow down the problem to one in which the mother and health professional are interested. For instance, to be able to apply her new knowledge, the mother will want to know the best method to use if the health professional advises that minimising house dust is effective. So you might ask 'what is the evidence for the effectiveness of measures to minimise the quantity of house dust mites on the severity of eczema?'
- Key words might be *allergy, dermatitis, eczema, mites, dust*. You might have other key words.

Examples of questions posed by the participants of the clinical effectiveness workshops

These are not given as examples that show particularly good or bad question formats, they are included here to show the range and variety of questions that individual participants in the workshops developed in conjunction with others in their practice or healthcare setting. These are the questions they used to search for the evidence and, when they found evidence, to interpret it and decide whether or not to put that evidence into practice.

- Is it cost-effective to screen all patients with diabetes for microalbuminuria?
- Is the routine use of potassium-sparing diuretics in association with loop diuretics clinically justifiable?
- How effective is involving healthcare support workers (as opposed to qualified nursing staff) in continence reviews?
- Is there any evidence that a vegetarian diet reduces the incidence of bowel cancer?
- Do raised triglyceride levels have an adverse effect on diabetics? If so, what treatment is advised?
- Is an optimal outcome for patients with breast cancer treated by lumpectomy dependent on follow-up in a secondary care clinic?
- Are there any dangers in using mouthwashes?
- Is there a link between a history of poor oral hygiene and decay in children's teeth?
- Should maintenance doses of thyroxine be given in accordance with blood levels of thyroxine or the presence of patients' symptoms?
- Do practice registers of patients with coronary heart disease improve patient care?
- Has any work been published on integrated care pathways in leukaemia?
- What is the outcome of patients developing pneumonia who have had pneumonia vaccine over the past five years?
- Are head lice best treated by malathion or permethrin?

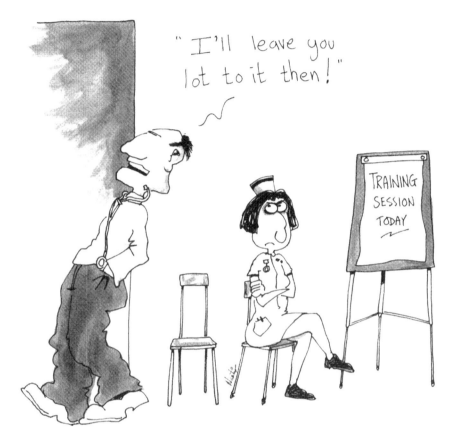

Clinical effectiveness is done best by involving the whole team.

Stage 2

Undertaking a literature search

The search strategy: think, search and appraise

A search for the best evidence follows the sequence of 'think, search and appraise'. This search strategy comprises:

- thinking about and defining a good specific question in consultation with all the staff who are involved in the question and affected by possible change(s)
- searching for and finding the best level of evidence by looking critically at the relevant publications obtained
- appraising and interpreting the evidence as applied to your question in relation to your situation.

Clinical effectiveness encompasses the whole cycle:

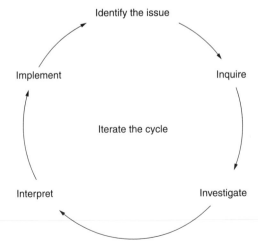

The clinical effectiveness cycle

The clinical effectiveness cycle.

It is tempting for health professionals who are pushed for time and hot on the scent of evidence with which to answer a question to jump straight from an idea to carrying out a search, instead of working through the steps with the necessary rigour. Cutting corners wastes time in the long run if you ask the wrong question, answer a different question to the one you intended, or become distracted by lots of interesting but irrelevant literature.

How long you spend and to what lengths you go with a search will depend on its purpose. If you were commissioned to undertake a major systematic review, you would spend many months searching every relevant database, hand searching through papers and journals, hunting up conference proceedings, trying personal contacts, translating non-English language papers, and generally leaving no stone unturned in the pursuit of published and unpublished studies. But as you are probably a busy clinician who just wants to find the best evidence for answering a question in practice, you should strictly limit your search as your resources are limited. You will probably be better off spending your precious time doing several searches for different topics than doing one exhaustive search on a single subject. So stop your search if you find a relevant systematic review of multiple, well-designed, randomised controlled trials in the Systematic Reviews section of the Cochrane Library. If there is no such systematic review move on to look for a review in the Database of Abstracts of Reviews of Effects (DARE). If no luck there try Medline, or EMBASE, or other specialist databases until you obtain the best possible level of evidence that you can find.

If you have not undertaken a search of the literature before, you would be well advised to book an individual session with your local healthcare librarian and to undertake a search in your health library if this is possible. You should be able to teach yourself from guidebooks, these notes, and trial and error, but a healthcare librarian is the person with the know-how about the best thesaurus terms and phrases to try with your search. You as a health professional will know about the validity, context and relevance of search words and phrases as applied to your question. Together, you as a clinician or other professional and the healthcare librarian make a strong search team.

Undertake a search

Before you start, *write down* the key words you want to use, putting them in order of importance. How many key words you enter at the first stage depends on how wide you expect your field of enquiry to be. If you key in *asthma*, you would expect to identify thousands more references to published papers than if you keyed in the name of a rare condition. So if you are searching within a broad topic area such as *asthma* you should prepare more potential words to narrow the field of your search for the few most relevant papers that will supply

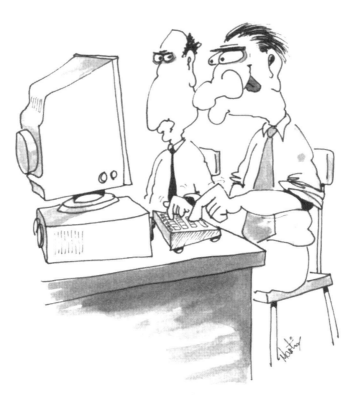

Book up with a healthcare librarian to help you search.

evidence to answer your original question. Refine your question prior to your search so that it is very focused and make sure that the key words are the most pertinent you can manage. Then you will spend less time on your search and have more chance of finding the most appropriate published evidence. So if you want to know more in the subject area of *asthma*, build your question carefully. Aim specifically at the purpose of the question and include the setting, the population under question, the intervention, the outcome and any other important details.

Using the Cochrane Library

Enter your most important key words first. Look at the different levels of evidence from the systematic reviews on the Cochrane Database of Systematic Reviews (CDSR) to controlled trials on the Cochrane Central Register of

Controlled Trials (CENTRAL) to the abstracts on the Database of Abstracts of Reviews of Effects (DARE). The hierarchy of evidence is explained further in the next section. You may find that you have access only to CDSR (see page 12).

It is likely that you will obtain only a small number of relevant-sounding systematic reviews, because this part of the Cochrane Library contains a relatively small number of specially written comprehensive reviews, rather than references to individual journal articles, as is the case in, for example, Medline. It is more likely that you will not find a relevant systematic review, but will identify many references to controlled trials. You should then modify your search by entering the first words again plus an extra key word that was your next choice in order of priority. If this does not refine your search enough, repeat the exercise, adding a fourth key word. When you have narrowed your search sufficiently, obtain copies of the original articles as appropriate so that you can critically appraise them yourself.

Do not assume that the contents of any paper published in a journal are valid, reliable or accurate, however reputable the journal. Mistakes may have been overlooked, studies reported might not be relevant to your own situation, or the results may not be generalisable to your question.

If your search on the Cochrane Library was unsuccessful, try another database with a larger number of individual references, such as Medline.

Using the Medline database

Because Medline contains an enormous number of references you will have to develop a very strict search strategy to narrow down your focus of enquiry. To search on Medline, a good starting point is to use the terms in its thesaurus, the Medical Subject Heading list (MeSH). There are over 17500 MeSH terms arranged as a tree structure with broad subject areas branching off and subdividing into narrower subject terms. If you use a word which is not a MeSH heading, Medline suggests an alternative. For instance if you type 'primary care', Medline suggests 'primary health care'. If you type 'cigarettes', 'smoking' is suggested.

Medline may be searched either by key word(s) in the title or abstract, or by selected headings from the MeSH list.

Entering one key word will often yield thousands of references, but a more selective search is possible by combining key words using 'and' and 'or' (these are called Boolean operators). To narrow the search further you can restrict the date range, the language the paper is written in, to 'Priority Journals' (an abridged list), or to 'human' as opposed to 'animal' research.

In a healthcare library, all you will need to do to access Medline or the Cochrane Library is to ask a member of staff. Your Athens password will also allow you to use your home (or any Internet-enabled) computer to search the databases.

There are two publications which give easy-to-follow practical details of undertaking a Medline search,[31,32] which you could consult if you are unfamiliar with Medline searching and want to read more about the process before having a go for yourself.

Hints for the use of Medline are:

*   click on a **Subject Heading** to view its position in the hierarchical 'Tree'
*   select the **Explode** box to retrieve references indexed under your selected MeSH heading plus all the more specific terms stemming from it
*   select the **Focus** box to limit your search to those documents in which your MeSH heading is considered to be the main point of the article.

You will learn most by having a go. You really cannot do anything wrong that you are not able to put right by retracing your steps.

The hierarchy of evidence

The table below shows one of the common ways of grading the evidence ranging from level I, which is the most robust evidence, to level V, based on the opinions of experts in the field.[28] There may not be any strong evidence in the literature for answering the question(s) you are posing.

Type	Evidence
I	Strong evidence from at least one systematic review of multiple, well-designed, randomised controlled trials
II	Strong evidence from at least one properly designed, randomised controlled trial of appropriate size
III	Evidence from well-designed trials without randomisation, single group pre–post, cohort, time series or matched case–control studies
IV	Evidence from well-designed non-experimental studies from more than one centre or research group
V	Opinions of respected authorities, based on clinical evidence, descriptive studies or reports of expert committees

The most valid types of research for extracting evidence about clinical effectiveness are randomised controlled trials, followed by controlled trials not using randomisation, then uncontrolled trials and, less reliably, observational studies. A systematic review of several randomised controlled trials of all known studies is better than a review of some studies, which in turn is better than a case study. You should start to search for the best evidence and, if you do not find it, work down the hierarchy.

If there is no reliable evidence to be found after searching the Cochrane Library, Medline and other relevant databases, you should then move on to look for any expert consensus agreements by multidisciplinary groups.

Be realistic – try to find one or a few key reviews rather than get bogged down in a plethora of papers. Clinical effectiveness is a tool for keeping up to date, enhancing your clinical practice, and retaining your professional interest – spending too much time pursuing it may be counterproductive.

> 'Most of my problems either have no answer or else the answer is worse than the problem.'

Examples

Example of literature search using problem 1 described previously

Question: What is the evidence for the effectiveness of a health professional advising a smoker to stop smoking?

Key words: *health education, smoking, primary healthcare, general practice*

The search used the MeSH headings *health education, smoking, primary health care, family practice* combined in the following way:

Advanced Search:

MEDLINE - 1950 to date (MEZZ)

(run saved search) (limit) (repeat) (remove duplicates) (split) (email) (save search) (create alert)

Search history:

No.	Database	Search term	Info added since	Results		
1	MEDLINE - 1950 to date	health-education#	48 months	17860	show titles	rank
2	MEDLINE - 1950 to date	smoking.DE.	48 months	18501	show titles	rank
3	MEDLINE - 1950 to date	1 AND 2	48 months	730	show titles	rank
4	MEDLINE - 1950 to date	3 AND lg=en	48 months	589	show titles	rank
5	MEDLINE - 1950 to date	primary-health-care#	48 months	11834	show titles	rank
6	MEDLINE - 1950 to date	family-practice	48 months	9146	show titles	rank
7	MEDLINE - 1950 to date	5 OR 6	48 months	19730	show titles	rank
8	MEDLINE - 1950 to date	4 AND 7	48 months	49	show titles	rank

hide | delete all search steps... | delete individual search steps...

Enter your search term(s): Search tips ☐ Thesaurus mapping

[   ] (whole document ◆)   (search)

ⓘ

Information added since: [   ] or: (48 months ◆)

Apple – Mac OS X

NB. Much better results will be obtained by combining individual MeSH terms than by attempting to ask a 'natural language' question such as 'Health education for smokers in general practice'. Doing this will simply 'confuse' the search engine.

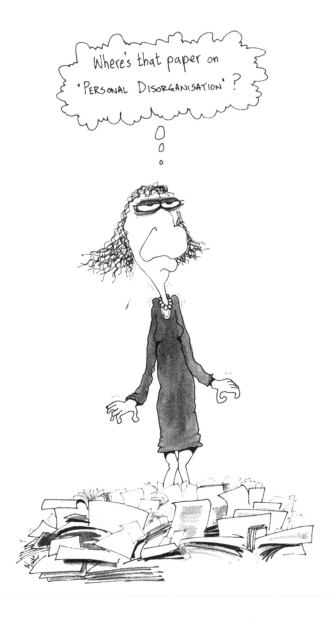

Use IT to ask a question and search for the evidence systematically.

The searcher has limited the search to recent papers published from 2002 onwards. Sets 1 and 2 show how many papers were referenced by Medline where *health education* and *smoking* were MeSH headings on the database. *Health education* was exploded (indicated by the #) so that the MeSH heading *patient education* would also be included in the search. *Smoking* was not exploded as the only other MeSH heading included would have been *marijuana smoking*, which was not relevant to this search.

Set 3 combines *health education* and *smoking* to find those 730 papers where both these MeSH headings appear. Set 4 confines the references obtained in the search to those 589 publications written in English. There are still too many abstracts to browse through to find relevant papers. So, to modify the search further and focus on the most relevant papers, the searcher added *primary health care* (exploded) in set 5 and *family practice* in set 6 to specify the setting in which *health education* and *smoking* were of interest. The MeSH heading *primary health care* has several branches and that is why the searcher has 'exploded' it in set 5 so that none of the branches are missed; but *family practice* is at the end of a branch and has therefore not been 'exploded'. Keying in *primary health care* or *family practice* found 19 730 papers, and many publications would have been missed if only one of these MeSH headings had been used.

By combining sets 4 and 7 (that is, looking for papers in English that have MeSH headings *health education* and *smoking* and *primary health care* or *family practice*), references were found to 49 papers. It is realistic to scroll through this number of abstracts to look for relevant publications. So the search could stop here if enough relevant material has been identified.

A search may be narrowed further by introducing the word 'not' to exclude unwanted aspects of a topic, or broadened by looking for other, related MeSH headings that appear elsewhere in the 'Tree'. Interestingly, *smoking cessation*, which is a very important MeSH heading in this search, is not included in the exploded MeSH heading *smoking*, and must be searched for separately.

An experienced healthcare librarian is an invaluable guide for a novice searcher. Besides knowing alternative MeSH headings such as *family practice* and *primary health care* as already described, the librarian will be able to advise on which databases are most appropriate for your search.

Example of literature search using problem 2 described previously

Question: What is the evidence for the effectiveness of measures to minimise numbers of house dust mites on the severity of eczema?

Key words: *allergy, dermatitis, eczema, mites, dust*

Cochrane Library 2006, Issue 2

Entering the words *eczema* or *dermatitis* and adding *mite** (using the * after mite means that any characters after the * are also searched for (in this case 'mites')), 764 references are found for *mite**, 2563 with the key word *dermatitis*, and 1020 for *eczema*. Using a combination of *dermatitis* or *eczema*, 3106 'hits' are scored; adding *mite** at this point gives 92 'hits' – 22 systematic reviews (CDSR), one abstract of reviews (DARE) and 68 references to controlled trials (CENTRAL), of which several seem appropriate, including:

- Gutgesell C, Heise S, Seubert S *et al*. Double-blind placebo-controlled house dust mite control measures in adult patients with atopic dermatitis. *Br J Dermatol* 2001; **145**: 70–4.
- Tan BB, Weald D, Strickland I *et al*. Double-blind controlled trial of effect of house-dust mite allergen avoidance on atopic dermatitis. *The Lancet* 1996; **347**: 15–18.
- Friedmann PS, Tan BB. Mite elimination – clinical effect on eczema. *Allergy* 1998; **53**(48 Suppl): 97–100.
- Hide DW, Matthews S, Matthews L *et al*. Effect of allergen avoidance in infancy on allergic manifestations at age two years. *J Allergy Clin Immunol* 1994; **93**: 842–6.

A 'belt and braces' technique makes sure you do not miss anything and you might key in *dust* instead of *mite*. This minimises your chances of missing any paper relating to *house dust*.

Cochrane Library

Medline database

No.	Database	Search term	Info added since	Results		
1	MEDLINE - 1950 to date	dermatitis#	unrestricted	64027	show titles	rank
2	MEDLINE - 1950 to date	mites#	unrestricted	10462	show titles	rank
3	MEDLINE - 1950 to date	1 AND 2	unrestricted	612	show titles	rank
4	MEDLINE - 1950 to date	3 AND lg=en	unrestricted	486	show titles	rank
5	MEDLINE - 1950 to date	4 NOT animals.DE.	unrestricted	80	show titles	rank
7	MEDLINE - 1950 to date	5	various	34	show titles	rank

Exploding the MeSH term *dermatitis* in set 1 ensures that all papers are identified where *any* type of eczema or *any* type of dermatitis is used as a MeSH term.

Adding the exploded MeSH term *mites* in set 2 and combining with set 1 using 'and' found 612 papers. Limiting to English language, papers added in the last four years, and excluding animal studies, reduced the set to 34 papers. Excluding 'animals' often gives better results than limiting to 'documents relating to humans', as the indexers frequently forget to use the 'human' check tag. Adding the MeSH term *dust* to further refine the search would not have been a good decision in this case, even though it might seem a logical thing to try. Many relevant papers have been indexed under *mites* but not *dust*. Only by experimenting and comparing the results of different strategies will you find the best one to suit each question. It is usually better to scan through a set of titles (so long as there are less than, say, 100) than risk missing important papers by trying to over-refine your search strategy. On the other hand, if few hits are being scored, it makes sense to broaden your MeSH strategy by also searching for words that you would expect to appear in the title or abstract of relevant papers. This will often find extra hits that have not been indexed using the most obvious MeSH headings. It will also pick up papers recently added to the database that have yet to be assigned thesaurus headings by the indexers.

'Focusing' a search is something that you should try only after finding that too many hits are being scored and that too many of those are not relevant to answering your question. It is important to remember that Medline is not a full-text database, so your search will not find words in the main body of the text, only in the title or abstract. In this example, the second 'hit' was the controlled trial by Gutgesell *et al.*, which was found in the Cochrane Library search, and several other relevant papers were also listed.

It is a good idea to print out the results of your search before you leave the screen, making concurrent notes on the paper print-out to remind you of the stages of your search, otherwise it will be a meaningless jumble at the end.

It is also possible to save your search strategy and edit it before printing if it needs 'tidying up'. Once saved, your strategy can be run at intervals to check for recently added papers.

Example of search using one of the workshop participant's questions

Question: Is it cost-effective to screen all patients with diabetes for micro-albuminuria?

Key words: *microalbuminuria, diabetes mellitus, screening, cost-effectiveness*

Cochrane Library: 2006, Issue 2

Keying in *diabet** ensured that papers with the words *diabetic* or *diabetes* were all included.

Similarly the key word *microalbumin** ensured that words with slightly different endings were all included. Browsing through the MeSH headings for *diabet** in the Cochrane Library reveals many specific types of diabetes in the thesaurus. Keying in *diabet** found 12 990 references, while *diabetes* found 11 097 references.

There was a total of 435 'hits' from searching on *microalbumin** and *diabet** in the Cochrane Library. Three were 'hits' on the Cochrane Database of Systematic Reviews (CDSR), one of which had been withdrawn for being out of date. There were references to 422 controlled trials in the Cochrane Central Register of Controlled Trials (CENTRAL) and five 'hits' on the Database of Abstracts of Reviews of Effects (DARE). Four 'economic evaluations' and one 'technology assessment' made up the total.

Modifying the search by adding the term *screen** reduced the number of controlled trials to 22 with one review in the CDSR.

The NHS Economic Evaluation Database (NHSEED) produced two 'hits' of which the following paper was particularly relevant:

- Le Floch JP, Charles MA, Philippon C, Perlemuter L. Cost-effectiveness of screening for microalbuminuria using immunochemical dipstick tests or laboratory assays in diabetic patients. *Diabet Med* 1994; **11**: 349–56.

Medline search: 1999 to date

The word *microalbuminuria* did not exist in the MeSH index – *albuminuria* was the nearest match. Keying in *diabetes* gave a selection of search words in the MeSH index; the searcher chose to select and explode *diabetes mellitus*. Keying in the word *screening* gave *mass screening* at the top of a list of suggested terms.

The screenshot below shows the results of the search on Medline for evidence to answer the same question:

The $ sign on Medline is equivalent to the * on the Cochrane Library: it allows a textword search to find the root word *screen*, plus *screens*, *screened* or *screening*, without having to key in those words separately. Several papers are retrieved on this search that have the word *screening* in their titles, but that have not been indexed under the MeSH term *mass screening*. This illustrates the importance of not relying solely on the indexers for complete accuracy or consistency.

Coincidentally, the healthcare librarian helping with this search remembered seeing a relevant paper in the local area's postgraduate journal:

- Davies S. Microalbuminuria. *Mid Med* 1997; **20**: 67–9.

This was a very helpful paper in a journal not indexed on either Cochrane or Medline, being part of the 'grey' literature (material either not published conventionally or indexed by a major database and thus difficult to identify). It was consistent with level V in the hierarchy of evidence, describing the opinion of a local well-informed expert who stated that 'microalbuminuria has been identified as the strongest predictor of diabetic nephropathy, with 80–90% of affected patients going on to develop this problem' and recommended annual screening of diabetic patients aged 12–70 years for microalbuminuria. This article cited four other relevant references, all of which were published before 1999, and had therefore been missed in this Medline search, which had been limited to published papers from 1999 onwards.

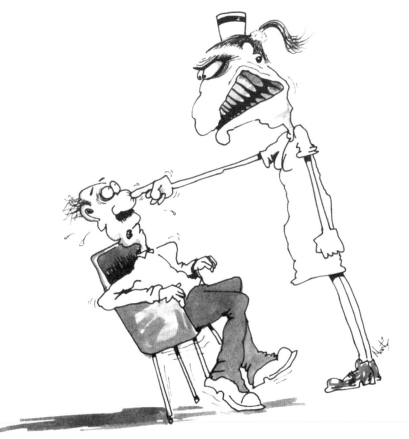

Information is power!

As a result of the evidence gained from the search, the workshop participant who posed this question instituted routine testing of patients with diabetes for microalbuminuria in the practice protocol.

Example of search using a second workshop participant's question

Question: Is an optimal outcome for patients with breast cancer treated by lumpectomy dependent on follow-up in a secondary care clinic, or is GP follow-up equally effective?

Key words: *breast cancer, lumpectomy, follow-up*

Cochrane Library: 2006, Issue 2

The MeSH term *breast neoplasms* identified 4959 references. As the MeSH term might not identify all controlled trials, *breast neoplasm** was searched as a textword and produced 5713 references. In order to be comprehensive, *breast cancer* was added and produced 9392 references. Combining the three searches above using the operator 'or' produced 9985 references (set 4).

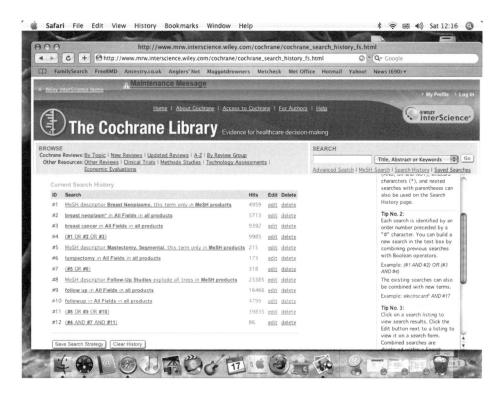

The MeSH term *mastectomy-segmental* was entered and produced 215 references. Entering *lumpectomy* as a textword identified 173 references and combining these two using the operator 'or' gave 318 (set 7). The MeSH term *follow-up studies* gave 23 385 references and textword *follow up* or *followup* produced 21 265. Combining these three using the operator 'or' gave 39 835 references (set 11). Finally, combining sets 4, 7 and 11 using the operator 'and' gave 86 references.

These included 72 'hits' on CENTRAL, three reviews on DARE, three hits on the NHS Economic Evaluation Database (NHSEED) and seven hits on the CDSR. One of these seven came to the conclusion that outcome for these women was not dependent on follow-up in a secondary care clinic: follow-up by a general practitioner seemed to be equally effective. In this example, a satisfactory answer was obtained from the Cochrane Library, as this systematic review cited all the papers that would have been retrieved by searching Medline and other databases. Knowing when to stop searching is an important part of practising clinical effectiveness! The paper in question is:

- Rojas MP, Telaro E, Russo A *et al*. Follow-up strategies for women treated for early breast cancer. The Cochrane Database of Systematic Reviews 2000, Issue 4, Art No.: CD001768.

It is important not to narrow your search too much at the beginning, and thus restrict yourself unnecessarily and risk missing papers that may have been indexed in a slightly different way.

Searching by yourself

Now you do it – work through an example by yourself.

1 Take any one (or all) of the four problems which interests you most – whether health education on smoking is worth doing, whether possible improvement in a child's eczema warrants the effort involved in minimising house dust at home, whether it is cost-effective to screen all people with diabetes for microalbuminuria, or whether patients who have had a lumpectomy for breast cancer are best followed up in secondary care. Adapt the problem(s) to your own circumstances. The idea of this exercise is that you will run a search on a similar question (or questions) to the ones already described so that you can follow the procedures laid out in this book for guidance, but adapted to your own situation so that it is more relevant to you. Conducting your own version of the search will give you more

confidence that you can do a literature search yourself. Write in your own words what your perspective of the problem is:

2 Frame the words of your question to address that problem – the words you use in the question should vary from any presented in this book as the angle of the problem and the focus of the question should relate to your own circumstances. Write in your own words what the question is:

3 Choose up to five key words and put them in order of priority:

4 Undertake a search for the evidence to answer that problem. If possible go to your health library and book time with a healthcare librarian who can help and advise you if necessary. Use the Cochrane Library first and then Medline.

Photocopy pages 43–45 if you undertake this exercise for more than one example question.

Cochrane search

- Write down how you will use your key words to search the Cochrane Library. Which one, two or three words will you key in first? Then, which words will you add, and in what order, to narrow the focus of your search?

- How did the search go? How many 'hits' did you obtain from the Cochrane Library?
  - systematic reviews on the Cochrane Database of Systematic Reviews (CDSR):
    (i) number of reviews =
    (ii) number of protocols =
  - controlled trials on the Cochrane Central Register of Controlled Trials (CENTRAL) =

    – abstracts on the Database of Abstracts of Reviews of Effects (DARE) =

- Print off up to five references that seem relevant to your question, so that you can obtain the original papers if you should wish to. Print off the abstracts if you have the facilities to do so.

Medline search

- Write down how you will use your key words to search the Medline database. Which one, two or three words will you key in first? Then, which words will you add, and in what order, to narrow the focus of your search?

- Begin your search and key the words in, exploding, combining and modifying the search according to the order of key words you have just specified and the numbers of papers you obtain at each stage. Go back to the instructions about using Medline and work through the examples and helpful suggestions if you have difficulties doing your own search.

- How did the search go? Print off your search strategy, to provide a record of the separate stages of your search. If you cannot print the strategy, copy it down in the table below under the headings 'Set', 'Search' and 'Results'.

Set	Search	Results
1		

- When you get down to fewer than 100 or so articles, scroll through the abstracts on the screen and print off the details of the ones that seem most relevant.

- If you have still not obtained any relevant evidence, you have a choice of trying other databases, or following up references given in papers with content nearest to your field of enquiry, or contacting experts named as authors or investigators to find out if there is work in press or other publications you have missed, or any other pertinent information. If you already know of one relevant paper, try to find the Medline entry for it by searching under the author's name and combining it with a search for words in the title. When you have found it, examine the full record to see what MeSH terms the indexers have used. This may give you some ideas for other terms to search under.

You should not expect to find exactly the same results as in the examples given earlier, as not only will you have modified the problem, the linked question and the search strategy to fit your own circumstances, but the details of publications held on the Cochrane and Medline databases will have been added to over time.

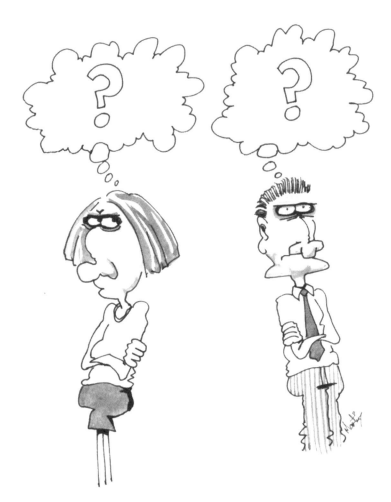

Choose a question that is important to you and your colleagues at work and where changes in practice will be possible.

Stage 3

Frame your own question and search for the evidence

Now that you have learned the theory behind doing a search and have seen how other health professionals like you have framed their questions and searched for the evidence, you should be ready to shape your own question and find the best available evidence that exists.

1 Think about a problem at work which you consider would be an appropriate topic for this exercise. Consult others at work; do they think it is a problem too? Is it an important issue for them and do they think you would be spending your time wisely searching for evidence about best practice? Is there likely to be a change that you could make which would bring benefits to you, colleagues or patients, or result in a saving of resources? As this book is considering how to improve clinical effectiveness you should choose a clinical topic in this instance, but another time you might choose to search for evidence on a management issue. What is the problem you have chosen to investigate? Write it down here:

Who else did you consult before deciding on this problem?

What sort of changes at work do you have in mind that might be possible to put into action, depending on what evidence you find?

2 Frame the words of your question which addresses that problem. Build up the question as described previously, being as specific as possible, but not so specific that you narrow your field of enquiry and eliminate possible options that might be appropriate, such as novel types of intervention. Include the

purpose of the question, what it is about, the setting, the population and the outcome(s). Write in your own words what the question is:

Are there any subsidiary questions?

Have you discussed the question with anyone else? If so, with whom?

3 Choose up to five key words and put them in order of priority:

Are you satisfied that these key words reflect all the essential ingredients of your original problem and capture the essence of the question?

4 Undertake a search for the evidence to answer the question. If possible go to your health library and book time with a healthcare librarian who can help and advise you if necessary. Try the Cochrane Library first and then Medline.

Cochrane search

- Write down how you will use your key words to search the Cochrane Library. Which one, two or three words will you key in first? Then, which words will you add, and in what order, to narrow the focus of your search?

- How did the search go? How many 'hits' did you obtain from the Cochrane Library?
  - systematic reviews on the Cochrane Database of Systematic Reviews (CDSR):
    (i) number of reviews =
    (ii) number of protocols =
  - controlled trials on the Cochrane Central Register of Controlled Trials (CENTRAL) =
  - abstracts on the Database of Abstracts of Reviews of Effects (DARE) =

- Print off up to five sets of details of articles that seem relevant to your question. Print off the abstracts of these articles if you are able to do so. Obtain copies of the original papers.

Medline search

- Write down how you will use your key words to search the Medline database. Which one, two or three words will you key in first? Then, which words will you add, and in what order, to narrow the focus of your search?

- Begin your search and key the words in, exploding, combining and modifying the search according to the order of key words you have just specified and the numbers of papers you obtain at each stage.

- How did the search go? Print off the results of the search in the same way as the screenshots given as examples earlier listed the stages of the search, the modifications and the numbers of papers identified from the key words. If you cannot print the results off the screen, copy them down here under the headings 'Set', 'Search' and 'Results'.

Set	Search	Results
1		

- When you get down to fewer than 100 or so articles, scroll through the abstracts on the screen and print off the details of the ones that seem most relevant.

- If you have still not obtained any relevant evidence you have a choice of trying other databases, or following up references given in papers with content nearest to your field of enquiry, or contacting experts named as authors or investigators to find out if there is work in press or other publications you have missed, or any other pertinent information. If you already know of one relevant paper, try to find the Medline entry for it by searching under the author's name and combining it with a search for words in the title. When you have found it, examine the full record to see what MeSH terms the indexers have used. This may give you some ideas for other terms to search under.

Dialog allows you to save your search strategy for re-running at a later date. Once a strategy has been saved, it can be edited and lines added, deleted or changed as your ideas develop.

Stage 4

Appraise the evidence

Now that you have extracted the publications that seem most relevant to your own question from your search, the next steps are to decide how much reliance you can put on their contents and how far you can extrapolate from those papers to your own circumstances. This will involve deciding whether the studies described in the papers were well conducted or flawed, whether the population and setting studied were similar enough to your own circumstances for the results to be generalisable to your population or setting, whether sufficient people or things were studied for the results to be representative of larger numbers, and how you will weigh one paper against another if they report conflicting results or conclusions.

Critical appraisal is the assessment of evidence by systematically reviewing its validity and results, and relevance to specific situations.

Critical appraisal:

- identifies the strengths and weaknesses of a research paper
- develops a better understanding of scientific principles and research methodology
- increases capability to understand to what extent published literature is applicable to other circumstances.

The meaning of different research methods and terms

Bias

Systematic deviation of the results from the true results due to the way(s) in which the study was carried out.

Confidence intervals

This describes the degree of confidence that can be placed on any statistical result. It describes the range of results from the subjects or things studied within which the investigator is 95% certain that the true population mean lies (the usual level of confidence chosen).

Confounder or confounding factor

A factor, other than the variables under study, which is not controlled for and which distorts the results causing a spurious association.

Controlled trial

As for a randomised controlled trial (see relevant entry) without the randomisation element.

A controlled trial detects associations between an intervention and an outcome but does not rule out the possibility that the association was caused by an unrecognised third factor linking both the intervention and the outcome.

Controls

The subjects in a (randomised) controlled trial who are (randomly) allocated to receive either placebo, no treatment or the standard treatment.

Cost-effectiveness analysis (CEA)

Compares the effectiveness of two interventions with the same treatment objectives. Competing interventions are compared in terms of costs per unit of consequence. Consequences may vary but are measured in monetary terms.

Cost–benefit analysis (CBA)

Compares the incremental costs and benefits of a programme. Measures both costs and benefits in monetary values and calculates net monetary gains or losses (presented as a cost–benefit ratio).

Cost-minimisation analysis (CMA)

Compares the costs of alternative treatments that have identical outcomes.

Cost–utility analysis (CUA)

Measures the effects of alternative interventions in terms of a combination of life expectancy and quality of life, using utility measures such as quality-adjusted life-years (QALYs), and may present relative costs per QALY.

Efficacy

The extent to which an intervention produces a beneficial result under ideal conditions. Preferably based on a randomised controlled trial (RCT).

Effectiveness

The extent to which an intervention does what it is intended to do for a defined population.

Hawthorne effect

The influence of knowledge of the study on behaviour. The effect of being in a study on the persons being studied.

Incidence

The numbers or proportion of new cases of a disease or condition occurring within a population over a given period of time.

Intention to treat analysis

This is a quantitative estimate of the benefit of a therapy in the population being studied derived from comparing control and treatment groups.

Numbers needed to treat (NNT) are being cited in published papers increasingly commonly. You need to know the characteristics of the population being studied, the disease and its severity, the treatment and its duration, the comparator and the outcomes.

Meta-analysis

This is a method of combining two or more studies to obtain information about larger numbers of subjects. Inclusion criteria should be clearly stated in the method to enable different studies to be considered together. It should appear reasonable to treat the sum of the different studies as one whole and that like is being combined with like.

Observational study

There are several types of study where the subjects are observed over time and the experiences are recorded or reported.

A cohort study is one where two similar groups of people who do not have the disease or condition under study are observed prospectively over a predetermined period to see the effects of one group being exposed to an already established suspected risk factor (such as cigarette smoking) and the other group not being so exposed.

A cross-sectional survey gathers information about subjects or things in a study population at one point in time or over a relatively short period.

Odds ratio (OR)

A measure of treatment effectiveness. The probability of an event happening as opposed to it not happening. An OR of 1 means that the effects of treatment are no different from no treatment. If the OR is greater than (or less than) 1, it means that the effects of treatment are more (or less) than those of the control group.

Placebo

An inert substance that is given to control subjects in trials.

Power

Sample sizes should be calculated before the study design is finalised to determine the numbers needed to be likely to detect a sufficient effect from the study intervention, so as to be sure that the effect did not occur by chance alone. The power calculation predicts the number that needs to be studied to detect an effect at least at the level of 95% significance. This is the level of certainty that is equal to or less than a one in 20 risk that the effect occurred by chance and was not due to an intervention or event being studied.

Prevalence

The proportion of 'cases' within a specified population at a given time.

Probability

Probabilities are often written as p values in published reports, where p stands for probability. It is a measure of how likely an outcome is. This lies between 0 (where an event will never happen) and 1.0 (where it will definitely occur).

The p value is a guide to the likelihood that the outcome measured occurred by chance or was due to the intervention or event that the study was designed to measure.

A significant p value is one where the likelihood is that the effect or outcome occurred as a result of the intervention or event being studied, and did not occur by chance. The most common convention is to decide arbitrarily on a one in 20 risk of being wrong about the direct causal relationship between the intervention or event and the outcome; that is, the risk that the outcome occurred by chance. This can be described as '$p = 0.05$', 'at the 5% significance level' or as a '5 in 100 probability' that the outcome occurred by chance. If written as '$p < 0.05$' there is less than a 5 in 100 risk of the outcome having happened by chance. Smaller p values give increased confidence in the test results; for example $p < 0.001$ indicates that the probability that the outcome occurred by chance is less than one in a thousand. The level of significance the investigators choose should depend on the importance of being right about the intervention/outcome relationship, and the numbers in the populations being studied.

Sometimes investigators get carried away, testing every bit of data in their study to see if they can dredge up some significant results. This is very bad practice because even a short questionnaire can yield hundreds of combinations of possibilities if each question has several alternative categories of answer, for example age might be subdivided into nine decades. If a significance test was applied to all the possible combinations of answers looking for potential links and 200 tests of significance were tried, for example, you would expect ten tests erroneously to indicate statistical significance where the outcome(s) had occurred by chance (that is, a 5 in 100 risk $\times$ 2 = 10). So the arbitrary $p < 0.05$ test of assumed significance is not cut-and-dried proof that an outcome is directly attributable to an intervention – it is just a good indicator of significance.

Publication bias

Results are more likely to be published if the results are positive rather than negative. Thus, it may appear that treatments have more positive results than is actually the case.

Randomised controlled trial (RCT)

Randomisation is necessary to minimise and, hopefully, eliminate selection bias. This is the type of study design which is most likely to give you a true result because only one section of the subjects or things in the trial are exposed to the intervention or factor being studied. The subjects or things are randomly allocated either to the group exposed to the intervention or to the control group, who are not intentionally exposed to that intervention. The experiences and outcomes of both groups are compared to see if they are significantly different according to statistical tests. Sometimes the design includes more than two comparative groups.

Using the randomised controlled trial method distributes unsuspected biological variables equally between the two groups, as well as any other external factors of which you are unaware. Both the subject and control groups will be exposed to these unrecognised external influences (called confounding factors) and any differences in outcomes between the two groups should be attributable to the intervention being studied.

When the term 'randomised' is stated there should be some information in the method as to how this randomisation process was carried out to minimise any external influences from interfering with the random allocation of subjects or things to different arms of the study.

If a trial is 'double blind', neither the clinician/investigator giving the treatment or analysing the results, nor the person receiving it, should know whether they are in the treatment or the control group. In a 'single' blind study, either the clinician or the subject knows what treatment the subject is receiving.

Relative risk

Relative risk is calculated by taking the ratio between two measures of risk. If there is no difference between two groups the risk ratio is '1', as the risks in each group are the same. A risk ratio greater than '1' shows the outcome in the study group to be better than that for controls.

The risk ratio is the proportion of the group at risk in one group divided by the proportion at risk in a second group. The risk ratio is a measure of relative risk.

Reliability

A reliable method is one which produces repeatable results.

Sensitivity of test

The true positive rate of a diagnostic test, that is, how often the test misses people with the disease.

Sensitivity analysis

Tests the robustness of the results of an economic analysis by varying the underlying assumptions around which there is uncertainty.

Specificity of test

The true negative rate of a diagnostic test, that is, how often the test indicates people as having the disease when they do not.

Statistically significant

By convention taken to be at the 5% level ($p < 0.05$). This means that the observed result would occur by chance in only one in 20 cases (*see* Probability).

Systematic review

Systematic reviews of randomised controlled trials provide the highest level of evidence of the effectiveness of treatments – preventative, therapeutic and rehabilitatory treatments (as described in the section on hierarchy of evidence, pp 32–3).

Validity

A valid method is one which measures what it sets out to measure.

Reading a paper

Reading and evaluating a paper is mainly about applying common sense. Traditionally, critical appraisal of the literature has been made to seem like a difficult science for the elite, rather than a basic skill that any health professional can readily learn and apply to their own situation.

If you read the summary of a research study overleaf and answer the questions, you will soon discover for yourself some of the common flaws in published studies, sometimes even those in respected peer-reviewed journals where the mistakes were not noted by the researchers or publication team.

In general you should consider whether:

- the paper is relevant to your own practice
- the research question is well defined
- any definitions are unambiguous
- the aim(s) and/or objective(s) of the study are clearly stated
- the design and methodology are appropriate for the aim(s) of the study
- the measuring instruments seem to be reliable; that is, different observers at different points in time would arrive at the same outcome
- the measuring instruments seem to be valid; that is, the investigator is actually measuring that which she/he intends to measure
- the sampling method is clear
- the results relate to the aim(s) and objective(s) of the study
- the results seem to be robust and justifiable
- the results can be generalised to your own circumstances
- there are any biases in the method of the study
- there are biases in the results, such as non-reporting of drop-outs from the study
- the conclusion is valid
- you have any other concerns about the study.

Specifically you should look at:

- where the study was done and who are the authors
- the study design: how were the subjects and controls selected, were they randomised and if so how, what were the outcome measures, were the outcome measures clinically relevant, are the sample numbers appropriate?

- the results: are the numbers of drop-outs and non-respondents reported, are all subjects accounted for, is the statistical analysis explained, are the results clearly presented?
- the discussion and conclusions: does the report describe the study's limitations, are the conclusions supported by the results?

Critical appraisal of a published paper or report of a study

1 The aim(s) and /or objective(s) of the study should be stated clearly.

- The aim should state the purpose of the study succinctly and specifically. It should be set in the context of information that is already known from previously published literature.
- The reasons for, and need to carry out, the study should be justified in the introduction of the paper.
- There should be a clear route built up from the aim to the conclusion flowing from the explanation of why a particular study design, population and setting were selected, to the results reported, the discussion and interpretation, and final conclusion(s).

2 The methodology should be appropriate for the aim(s) of the study.

- Quantitative and qualitative design techniques are complementary. A good quantitative survey will be based on prior qualitative work to determine what are appropriate questions to ask in the questionnaire or interview schedule. A randomised controlled trial may be a gold standard quantitative study design, but a qualitative method will most probably be needed to report people's observations, reflections and judgements.
- As a generalisation, prospective recording is more likely to be accurate than retrospective recall.
- A sample of a population should be selected for study which is as representative as possible of the whole population.
- A setting should be chosen for a study which is as representative as possible of the setting of the total population to which the results of the study will be extrapolated.
- The sample size should be justified by a *power calculation* determined prior to starting the study based on the expected findings.
- There should be a method for increasing the response rate to as near as possible an ideal of 100% of the subjects included in the study.
- Details of any measurement or intervention should be as specific as possible, and transparently valid and reliable.

- A good study design will include a method to validate the questionnaire, rating scale or results obtained.
- It is always a bonus to see an original questionnaire, even if only in an abbreviated form, to be able to judge for yourself the validity of the questions used in the study.
- The statistical methods should be described so that when the results are reported readers can check the statistical calculations and understand how the results were derived from the original data, if they wish.

3 The results should be robust, justified and related to the objectives of the study.

- The results should be simple to understand. It should be obvious where the results have come from and they should not seem to have been plucked out of thin air. Graphs and tables help to avoid strings of numbers and percentages.
- Statistically significant results should be presented in a conventional way or explained with full references if less well-known statistical tests are used.
- Percentages should normally add up to 100% and if they do not there should be some explanation to account for the missing numbers. It should be clear where and whether subjects have not sent back the questionnaire, have left a particular question blank or given a 'don't know' response.
- If the results obtained from the subjects are fairly crude, such as when people are asked to estimate their answers or recall happenings in the distant past, the result should be given as whole numbers or to one decimal place, rather than to several decimal places, which might look more scientific to the casual reader.
- The written contents of a research paper should be in their correct places. Bits of method should not crop up afresh in the results, nor should discussion be interspersed in the results. The flow of the paper should be logical and build up to a justifiable conclusion. Anything otherwise is confusion and muddle.
- A low response rate may mean that the results from the sample of the population studied are not likely to be representative of the whole population. The further you regress from a 100% response rate the more likely it is that you have missed people or things that would give your results a different slant. As a very rough guide, a response rate of 70% seems generally to be regarded as reasonable for a topic where the results are not going to have dire consequences if they are wrong. But if the study was a trial of drug therapy where people's lives might be at stake if the research results and conclusions were wrong, anything less than a 100% response rate might be unacceptable.

4 Any biases in the design and execution of the study should be minimised
   and their likely influences acknowledged and explained.

   • Good response rates are important because responders may have
      different characteristics from those of non-responders.
   • There may be confounding factors present. These are so-far undetected
      influences that were not measured or recorded in the course of the study,
      which were actually wholly or partly responsible for causing the changes
      or results reported. There are often cultural changes with time outside
      the study and beyond the control of those undertaking the investigation.
      For instance, if a famous celebrity claimed benefits for a new treatment
      that was being studied, many more people would suddenly believe they
      had received the same benefits and the outcomes being studied at that
      time would be distorted. Opting for *randomised controlled trials* avoids the
      influence of confounding factors.
   • The potential and actual biases of the study should be openly described
      and their likely effects discussed in the Discussion section of the paper.
      Readers should then be able to make up their own minds about the
      relative importance of each bias on the results and how much the biases
      prejudice the extrapolation of the results to the readers' own situations.

5 Is the conclusion valid?

   • The conclusion is often found in the Discussion section of a paper when
      there is no separate Conclusion section.
   • The conclusions of the results should not hinge on probability test
      results. The significance of the results claimed should make sense from
      clinical and common sense perspectives too. For example, an interven-
      tion might claim that it is significantly better than another at increasing
      small children's height by 0.1 inches. But if, clinically, this difference is
      inconsequential, then the benefits of the treatment claiming to be
      superior are not proven by the positive significant result.
   • The conclusion(s) should not make any claims that have not been
      justified previously in the report of the study.
   • No new information should suddenly crop up in the conclusions that
      was not previously cited in the Method, Results or any other section.
   • It should be clear what the main findings mean and the implications for
      current practice or future developments.
   • The results of the current study should be compared and contrasted with
      others reported elsewhere, and any discrepancies interpreted and discussed.

6 Are there any other concerns about the study?

   • Conflicts of interest should be stated, such as the sponsorship of the
      study by a manufacturer of the medication tested in the study.

- Look for any omissions in any section of the report. Think whether the implications from any contrary results seem to have been considered in full or glossed over.

Examples

Critically appraise this example – a summary report of a research study.

1 An investigation of the use of sunscreens in the United Kingdom

Summary

Aim: To investigate the use of sunscreens in children.

Method: A postal questionnaire was sent out to all 942 members of Women's Institutes throughout the Scottish Isles, asking them about the frequency of the use of high-factor sunscreens applied to their children (please contact the author for a copy of the questionnaire). Questionnaires were anonymous to ensure confidentiality. An article was placed in the Women's Institute newsletter to prompt non-responders.

Results: 356 women replied (85% response rate; average age $56 \pm SD$ 16.4298 years). 290 stated that they bought factor 10 or higher sunscreen. 89 preferred the scent-free version ($p < 0.1$). 350 women thought that the government should subsidise the cost of sunscreens as they were too expensive ($p < 0.0001$). The presence of a melanoma should be treated as a criminal offence and the sufferer fined for not having used sufficient sunscreen, as a contribution to the costs of the ensuing NHS treatment.

Conclusion: If the government were to subsidise the cost of buying high-factor sunscreens, uptake would be increased and the frequency of melanomas or other skin cancers would fall.

Source of funding: Nibblea Suncreams.

Conflict of interest: None.

Chambers R. *J Evidence-Based Spoof* 1998; **3**: 12.

Consider the following challenges

Write down your answers then read the author's opinion below:

1   Are the aim(s) and/or objective(s) of the study clearly stated?
2   Is the methodology appropriate for the aim(s) of the study?

3 Do the results relate to the aims(s) and/or objective(s) of the study? Are the results robust and justified?
4 Are there any biases in the design and execution of the study?
5 Is the conclusion valid?
6 Are there any other concerns about the study?

Critique of the summary report: use of sunscreens in the United Kingdom

1 Are the aim(s) and/or objective(s) of the study clearly stated?

The aim is not very specific. If the focus of the conclusion on cost of sunscreens and the impact of sunscreens on the frequency of cancers was intended as the purpose of the study then the aim has been expressed incorrectly.

2 Is the methodology appropriate for the aim(s) of the study?

No, no, no! There is already confusion as the aim and conclusions are so far apart, but working on the premise of the aim stated in the summary of the study given:

- the population chosen for study is inappropriate as children of Women's Institute members probably range in age from 1 to 60 years old; this can be deduced from the subject's average age being 56 years and the standard deviation (SD) of 16.4 years, indicating that about two-thirds of the population studied are between ca. 40 and 72 years (that is, 56 – 16.4 years = $\sim$ 40 years to 56 + 16.4 years = 72 years)
- the Scottish Isles setting is in a part of the United Kingdom that would be expected to have relatively low amounts and strength of ultraviolet rays, and results from this setting cannot necessarily be generalised elsewhere
- members of Women's Institutes living in the Scottish Isles while the study was in progress had not necessarily lived there all their lives; so if the geographical area was important the mothers do not have uniform histories of where they lived when younger, and their children may have lived apart from their mothers at any time previously
- the age range of the children means that some mothers' reports will relate to children under the age of 18 years currently receiving modern types of high-factor sunscreens, and others will relate to middle-aged children who may or may not have had old-fashioned creams applied a varying number of years previously; high-factor sunscreens did not exist at the time the study began
- there is no logic in choosing Women's Institute members as the population group to be studied – it may introduce a further bias if it were shown that members were more likely to be part of a more affluent section of society than the population as a whole and therefore more

likely to take holidays abroad where the sunshine was more powerful and potentially damaging
- mothers' recall of the frequency of use of suncreams applied to children up to 50 years before is unlikely to be accurate
- anonymous questionnaires that do not bear a code number make chasing up of individual non-respondents impossible – an article placed in a newsletter is unlikely to be an effective method of encouraging non-responders to reply.

3 Do the results relate to the aim(s) and/or objective(s) of the study? Are the results robust and justified?

It is obvious that the results are inaccurate and meaningless. Also:

- the response rate was very low at 38% (356/942), not 85% as stated
- the results, such as the information about costs of sunscreens, are not related to the data that would have arisen from the study method described
- it is ridiculous to give the standard deviation (SD) to four decimal places when the average age is given as a whole number
- a probability of < 0.1 is not significant and no such conclusions can be drawn about a proportion of the population studied preferring the scent-free version
- results should be factual and not offer interpretations as here, where the government is encouraged to treat the presence of melanomas as a criminal offence
- the results cannot be generalised.

4 Are there any biases in the design and execution of the study?

The study is riddled with biases from start to finish. Many have been described already, such as:

- the nature of the population
- that retrospective recall of information is likely to be poor
- the poor response rate
- the changing nature of commercially available sunscreens over time throughout the study
- the fact that the conclusion does not relate to the rest of the study, which implies that the whole purpose of the study may have been to show that sunscreens should be subsidised and that the design and reporting of the study might be biased to that end.

5 Is the conclusion valid?

No it is not. It does not follow from the rest of the report and is not related to the original aim.

6   Are there are any other concerns about the study?

Although the author of this report states that there was no conflict of interest, the sponsorship of the study by a manufacturer of suncreams should alert readers to scrutinise the report even more carefully than usual for possible biases.

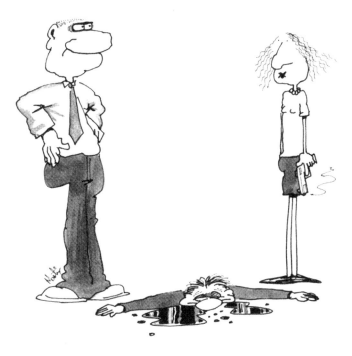

Remember that sometimes the evidence can be misleading.

2 An investigation of prisoners' health compared with that of the general population

Critically appraise this second example – an unpublished report of a research study. Answer the following challenges as before – write down your answers then read the author's opinion:

1   Are the aim(s) and/or objective(s) of the study clearly stated?
2   Is the methodology appropriate for the aim(s) of the study?

3 Do the results relate to the aims(s) and/or objective(s) of the study? Are the results robust and justified?
4 Are there any biases in the design and execution of the study?
5 Is the conclusion valid?
6 Are there any other concerns about the study?

Introduction: Recent work has shown that prisoners are disadvantaged in terms of their social background, their health status and the quality of healthcare they receive (Smith 1984; Walmsley *et al.* 1992). Research carried out in Bedford prison (Martin *et al.* 1984) found that prisoners had tended to neglect their health before reception into prison and 46% had active medical problems at admission.

Many of the people sent to prison have mental health problems. Gunn and others (1991) found that 37% of sentenced prisoners sampled from prisons in England and Wales had a psychiatric disorder, 2% of whom were suffering from a psychosis that was being inadequately treated and required transfer to hospital. A further 15% were thought to require additional treatment at the prison for their psychiatric problems.

The suicide rate among prisoners is several times that of their peers in the community and is rising disproportionately to the increase in the prison population (Dooley 1990). In 1992–93 (Wool 1994), 27 male prisoners committed suicide and in addition there were open verdicts on ten other males who died. The number of recorded incidents of self-injury is also rising steadily – 2612 prisoners were reported to have injured themselves on 3281 occasions in 1992–93 (Wool 1994).

A recent review of prisoners' physical health (Adam 1994) reported an increased incidence of alcohol problems, epilepsy, peptic ulceration, hypertension, hepatitis B infection, tuberculosis and self-neglect (skin infections, caries). Alcoholism is ten times more common among new prisoners than in the general community and 86% of new prisoners smoke (Martin *et al.* 1984).

This study set out to compare lifestyle habits of inmates in six prisons in the West Midlands with general population norms and measured prisoners' general health using the SF36 health measure (Jenkinson *et al.* 1993).

Method: Between 50 and 61 prisoners in each of the six prisons were surveyed between March and August 1994. Prisoners were interviewed in private rooms by the research associate. All prisoners thought to offer a potential security risk and those residing in punishment blocks were excluded from the study. Fifty prisoners were recruited in all establishments except one prison where 61 prisoners were chosen to allow sufficient sampling of the remand as well as the convicted men, and a second prison where 60 men were selected when two blocks of prisoners were demarcated for the study.

The method of selection varied according to individual prison procedures. In three prisons, clerical staff did not allow access to lists of prisoners' names and prisoners were recruited by a volunteer system. In the fourth prison all 60 inmates on education and physical education courses were interviewed. In the fifth and sixth prisons, every tenth inmate was selected from the list of inmates. Prisoners who refused or could not be interviewed were replaced by volunteers.

The interviews were conducted in a private room in which only the researcher and inmate were present, or a quiet corner of a large room. The inmate was assured that any information given was confidential to the research team and that a report would not identify any individual prisoners. All questions were asked by the interviewer so that literacy was not required.

The interviewer asked questions about lifestyle, and administered the SF36 survey form (Saudi Arabian version) (Ware and Sherbourne 1992).

The question schedule was piloted on ten prisoners before the main study began. Questions were amended accordingly. The prisoners participating in the pilot survey were excluded from the prison population selected for the survey.

A Minitab statistical package was used for processing the data and analysing the results.

Results: Thirty-six of the total 381 prisoners invited to be interviewed did not attend because they were unwilling, had appointments elsewhere, were thought by prison staff to be unsuitable for interview for security reasons, were confined to the punishment blocks or refused to be studied.

The mean ages of prisoners interviewed are shown in Table 1. All were convicted prisoners except 24 of the 61 surveyed in one prison, who were on remand.

Table 1: Age of prisoners interviewed in the six prisons studied

Prison code number	Mean age of subjects (standard deviation)*
P1 ($n = 61$)	18.2 (1.5)
P2 ($n = 60$)	16.1 (0.9)
P3 ($n = 50$)	32.4 (11.1)
P4 ($n = 50$)	27.4 (6.5)
P5 ($n = 50$)	32.1 (9.9)
P6 ($n = 50$)	19.7 (0.9)

* Age ranges have not been given so as to preserve prison anonymity.

Table 2 describes prisoners' smoking habits in prison. Smoking was as common among young offenders as older adults. Less than five per cent of prisoners who had previously not been smoking had started smoking during their time in prison. There was a slight tendency for smokers to report that they smoked more heavily since coming to prison.

Table 2:   Current smoking habits of inmates in the six prisons

Prison code number	Percentage of prisoners who were current smokers
P1 ($n = 61$)	90
P2 ($n = 60$)	82
P3 ($n = 50$)	82
P4 ($n = 50$)	88
P5 ($n = 50$)	60
P6 ($n = 50$)	90

The majority of inmates (91%) in all six prisons exercised on three days per week or more. Six per cent of prisoners never exercised in five of the six prisons. Forty-six per cent of prisoners interviewed reported that they exercised more during their time in prison compared to when they were 'outside', 15% thought the frequency was about the same and 38% thought they exercised less in prison.

All 321 prisoners who completed the questionnaire about lifestyle also answered the SF36 health survey. Table 3 gives the mean score for the eight variables of the SF36 and norms for a comparable group from the general population matched for age and sex, taken from Jenkinson *et al.* (1993). Prisoner means that were statistically different from general population norms are indicated in Table 3.

Mean SF36 scores for prisoners of all six prisons were significantly worse than the general population norms for social functioning ($p < 0.001$ in all cases), mental health ($p < 0.001$ in five out of six prisons, and $p < 0.05$ in P4) and pain dimensions; in five out of six prisons, inmates had mean SF36 scores that were significantly worse than age- and sex-matched norms for physical limitations and vitality.

Discussion: This survey proves that prisoners have worse health and wellbeing according to a comparison with the general public using the SF36 scale.

The volunteers used in place of those prisoners who refused or were not allowed to participate in the study were suitable replacements as the inter-viewer picked subjects who worked in the same workplace or lived in the same prison wings instead. The chocolate gratuity received by prisoners who had satisfied the interviewer's questions was not considered to have biased the results.

Prisoners' exercise habits compared favourably with those of doctors, where 22% have been found never to exercise and only 16% to exercise at least twice per week (Chambers 1992). Far more of the prisoner subjects smoked

Table 3: Mean scores for eight variables of SF36 for prisoners from the six prisons and norms for a comparable group matched for age and sex, taken from Jenkinson *et al.* (1993)

Prison code number	Physical function	Social function	Physical limits	Emotional limits	Mental health	Energy/ vitality	Pain	General health
P1								
Age/sex match	92.8	90.2	91.8	82.9	74.8	66.4	86.6	72.0
Prisoners	97.5*	78.9**	80.0**	77.0	65.3*	57.3**	75.4**	67.3
P2								
Age/sex match	92.8	90.2	91.8	82.9	74.8	66.4	86.6	72.0
Prisoners	97.1	81.6**	73.8**	81.7	63.5**	49.3**	75.3**	68.4
P3								
Age/sex match	91.9	90.4	90.4	85.4	75.5	64.7	85.9	73.9
Prisoners	91.8	70.7**	78.5**	66.6**	65.2**	54.7**	67.7**	68.5
P4								
Age/sex match	93.1	90.7	91.6	85.1	75.3	65.2	86.8	74.3
Prisoners	93.7	72.9**	85.5	74.6*	69.4*	60.5	72.2**	66.1*
P5								
Age/sex match	90.2	86.6	86.0	80.2	71.5	58.8	80.8	74.7
Prisoners	81.2**	64.9**	76.0*	58.5**	53.5**	42.3**	54.5**	63.6**
P6								
Age/sex match	92.8	90.2	91.8	82.9	74.8	66.4	86.6	72.0
Prisoners	96.3	76.7**	84.0*	86.0	66.6**	59.4*	77.9*	66.9

Prisoner means that are statistically significant in comparison with the group matched for age and sex are shown by *($p < 0.05$) or **($p < 0.001$).

compared to a third of adults in the general population (Health Education Authority 1989).

The SF36 scale is reliable, valid and acceptable. The number of statistically significant differences was startling compared to the general public's norms.

Conclusions: The general public is healthier than prisoners in the United Kingdom.

References for the paper:

- Adam S. *Learning Across the Walls: the prison service and the NHS.* London: King's Fund Centre; 1994.

- Chambers R. Health and lifestyle of general practitioners and teachers. *Occup Med* 1992; **42**: 69–78.
- Dooley E. Prison suicide in England and Wales, 1972–87. *Br J Psych* 1990; **156**: 40–5.
- Gunn J, Maden A, Swinton M. Treatment needs of prisoners with psychiatric disorders. *BMJ* 1991; **303**: 338–41.
- Health Education Authority. *Strategic Plan 1990–95*. London: Health Education Authority; 1989.
- Jenkinson C, Coulter A, Wright L. Short form 36 (SF36) health survey questionnaire: normative data for adults of working age. *BMJ* 1993; **306**: 1437–40.
- Martin E, Colebrook M, Gray A. Health of prisoners admitted to and discharged from Bedford prison. *BMJ* 1984; **289**: 965–7.
- Smith R. *Prison Health Care*. London: British Medical Association; 1984.
- Walmsley R, Howard L, White S. *National Prison Survey 1991*. London: HMSO; 1992.
- Ware JE, Sherbourne CD. The MOS 36-item short-form health survey (SF36) 1: conceptual framework and item selection. *Med Care* 1992; **30**: 473–83.
- Wool R. *Report of the Director of Health Care for Prisoners. April 1992–March 1993*. HM Prison Service; 1994.

Critique of the report: an investigation of how healthy prisoners are compared with the general population

This critique picks out main points and is not intended to be comprehensive. The report concerns a real study that was carried out by the author but has been adulterated to illustrate learning points.

1 Are the aim(s) and/or objective(s) of the study clearly stated?

Yes, they are stated at the end of the introduction. But the bulk of the material set out in the introduction refers to the mental health of prisoners, whereas the aims imply that the study is mainly concerned with prisoners' physical health.

2 Is the methodology appropriate for the aim(s) of the study?

- The use of an interviewer for questioning prisoners seems appropriate as a considerable number of prisoners might be expected to be illiterate.
- There is no power calculation or indication of whether 50 to 61 inmates from each prison were valid sample sizes.
- The Saudi Arabian version of the SF36 might be inappropriate for measuring the health of a British population.
- It was good that a pilot study was undertaken to test the questionnaire and that those subjects were excluded from the main study.

- There is insufficient detail about recruitment and selection of prisons and subjects, administration and contents of the questionnaire for another researcher to be able to repeat the study in the future.

3 Do the results relate to the aims(s) and/or objective(s) of the study? Are the results robust and justified?

- There is an error in that the first line gives the total number of prisoners as 381 whereas the tables and other text describe 321 prisoners being invited to interview. This might indicate either a simple error in the report or an attempt to disguise the numbers of prisoners refusing to be interviewed.
- The table giving the SF36 results (Table 3) is very complicated and difficult to understand.
- There is no indication of what statistical test was used to calculate statistical significance and probabilities.
- Percentages rather than actual numbers of prisoners exercising were given so that it is impossible for the reader to check that the percentages have been calculated accurately.
- Results on rows P1, P2 and P6 are the same.

4 Are there any biases in the design and execution of the study?

- There is no information about how the six prisons were selected nor how representative they were compared to others in the West Midlands or in the United Kingdom.
- The recruitment of prisoners by a mix of random selection and volunteers produced biased samples. The potential biases this created, if for example the volunteers were more health conscious, were not discussed anywhere in the paper.
- The prisoners' SF36 scores were compared with published norms for the general population. No account was taken of the likely different characteristics of prisoners with regard to previous level of education, literacy, occupational class, etc., and whether this might make comparison with average norms invalid.
- The method states that some prisoners were interviewed in a public room, throwing into doubt whether such interviewees would feel able to divulge sensitive information about themselves.
- There is no justification of why the SF36 was the scale chosen to measure general health of a prison population, nor whether it had ever been used for assessing prisoners before.
- Results for remand and convicted prisoners are mixed together with no indication of whether they are similar or why they are being combined.
- The 'chocolate gratuity' may have influenced prisoners in deciding to take part and in the answers they gave about their health.

- Comparison of prisoners' exercise habits with doctors and teachers does not make sense as they are such different populations.

5 Is the conclusion valid?

- No – the study has not proved that the general public are 'healthier' than prisoners. The results from prisoners in six prisons in one region in England cannot necessarily be extrapolated to the whole prison population of the United Kingdom. All the other types of potential biases to the results that are described above render such a conclusion invalid.
- The word 'healthier' has not been defined in the paper at all.

6 Are there any other concerns about the study?

- Information about chocolate rewards for completing the study is only admitted in the discussion and was omitted from the description of the method. Besides being wrongly placed, this raises suspicions about what else might have been omitted from the report.
- It is not clear why the researchers undertook such a study if they did not have officially approved access to prisoners' details.

So now critically appraise the report of a study you have identified from your search.

1 Are the aim(s) and/or objective(s) of the study clearly stated?
2 Is the design appropriate for fulfilling the aims – the population, the setting, the sampling technique, the type of study, the methods of measurement, avoidance of biases or confounding factors? Are all stages of the design described such that you could repeat the exact same study if you had a mind to do so?
3 Do the results relate to the aim(s) and/or objective(s) of the study? Are the results robust and justifiable? Can the results be generalised to your own circumstances? Are the results clear? Are there mistakes in the results?
4 Are there any biases in the design and execution of the study? Are they discussed in sufficient detail and are allowances made for their effects?
5 Are the conclusion(s) valid? What do they mean for your own practice?
6 Have you any other concerns about the study?

Critical appraisal of a qualitative research paper

Although qualitative research is not part of the hierarchy of evidence, it can provide a useful source of evidence. Qualitative research has been used extensively in the fields of nursing, allied health professionals (AHPs), mental health and the evaluation of the health service. Indeed, many nurses and AHPs searching for evidence in respect of their disciplines may find that while no quantitative research has been undertaken, there may be a number of published qualitative studies. Thus, it is essential that you are able to make a judgement about the quality of these types of studies as well. The following checklist and reminders about features you should consider is modified from Greenhalgh and Taylor (1997).[33]

1 Did the paper address an important clinical problem? Was the research question clearly formulated and defined?
   There should be a clear statement about why the research was done and the research question that was addressed.

2 Is a qualitative approach the best method of answering this research question?
   Qualitative research is useful for exploring beliefs, feelings and perceptions; for gaining a deeper understanding of an area; for exploring situations where little is known; for exploring sensitive issues; for gaining the 'whole picture'; and for allowing participants to speak for themselves. If this is what is being done, then a qualitative approach is almost certainly best. But think whether a quantitative approach, such as a randomised controlled trial (RCT), would have been more appropriate.

3 Is the setting/context for the research clear? How were the subjects selected? Is the sampling strategy described in detail? Is this strategy justified?
   Qualitative research is about exploring the beliefs and gaining a deeper understanding of the experiences of a particular group of people or individuals. The sample is therefore selected in order to include people from these groups. That is, people are chosen because they are part of that group, rather than being chosen at random or to represent the 'average' view.

4 Have the researcher's perspective, beliefs, experiences and background been taken into account?
   'Researcher' or 'observer' bias is important in qualitative research as the interviewer's background, knowledge, experience, beliefs, etc., may have an influence on the results of semi-structured interviews and focus groups. It is impossible to eliminate researcher bias, so the authors should address this problem by

discussing the researcher's perspective and how this might have influenced the interpretation of the results.

5 What data collection methods were used and are these described in detail?
Rigorous reporting of methods in articles about qualitative research is particularly important, as each study is unique in design and analysis. The methods tell the 'story' that is needed to interpret the results. Hoddinott and Pill (1997)[34] suggest that you should ask the following questions:

- *are the researchers' roles and qualifications clear?*
- *are interviewer details given?*
- *is the paper explicit about how respondents were recruited, who recruited them and how the research was explained to them?*
- *is it explicit about whether the interviewer was known to the respondents and how they were introduced?*
- *is the interview setting clearly stated?*
- *were methodological issues about the influence of the interviewer on the data addressed?*

6 What methods were used to analyse the data? What quality control measures were implemented? Was an attempt made to test the validity of the results? Was an attempt made to test the reliability of the results?
There are various different methods of analysing qualitative data, e.g. content analysis and grounded theory. You should look for evidence that the researcher has analysed the data in a systematic way. Do the authors state that the data, e.g. transcripts, field notes or audio tapes, are available for independent review? The authors should have looked for cases which contradict the developing theories. The data should have been independently analysed by another researcher or a second researcher should have repeated the analysis.

7 Are the results credible? Are the findings clinically important?
Use your common sense and ask 'Do the results seem sensible and believable? Will they matter in practice?' You should also look at whether the authors present sufficient original data, e.g. verbatim quotes, and whether these are indexed to subjects so that they could be traced back and checked.

8 What conclusions were made? Are the conclusions justified by the results?
In qualitative research the results and the discussion are not separate as in quantitative research, as the results are an interpretation of the data. You can look for evidence that the conclusions are 'grounded in evidence', i.e. that they flow from the findings, how comprehensible the explanations are, how well the analysis explains why people behave in the way they do, and how well the explanation fits with what is already known.

9 Can the findings be transferred to other clinical settings?
   Qualitative research is often criticised for only being applicable to the setting in which it was conducted. However, if true theoretical sampling rather than simply convenience sampling has been used, then the results are likely to be more transferable.

The checklist outlined above is not as all-encompassing or universally applicable as a checklist for critically appraising quantitative research, as qualitative research is 'by its very nature, non-standard, unconfined, and dependent on the subjective experience of both the researcher and the researched'.[33] This checklist sets some useful ground rules which may be enhanced by information given in other sources.[34–38]

Critically appraise a review

Now that you have learned to critically appraise a research report, try your hand at appraising a review. Refer back to the explanations about randomised controlled trials, probability, confidence limits or other scientific terms described in the earlier text if necessary. The same rules apply for carrying out a survey of all research about a topic as for individual research papers. The specific question being addressed must be stated explicitly, the subject population (relevant research reports) identified and accessed, appropriate information obtained in an unbiased fashion (by using specific criteria to identify which research reports should, and should not, be included in the review) and the final conclusions should relate to the evidence obtained from the research reports included in the review related back to the primary survey question.
   Look particularly for information in the review to reassure you of the following:

* The topic and purpose of the review are specified.
* The search methods used to find evidence relating to the question should be stated. The review of the literature should be comprehensive – reasonable efforts should have been made to identify and include relevant studies by consulting a range of databases and tracking down 'grey' material such as that in books, from conference proceedings, consensus statements or annual reports.
* The studies included in the review should be relevant and appropriate to the main subject or issue being addressed.
* Only similar data have been combined from different studies with similar subject characteristics, circumstances and methodologies. The methods used to combine the findings of the studies included in the review should be stated.

- There should be enough details about the subjects, populations, settings and other important factors for you to be able to decide whether the review's results and conclusions will be relevant to your particular circumstances.
- The criteria used to define whether or not a study was included in the overview should be stated clearly in the Methods section. The researchers should have adhered to those explicit inclusion criteria, avoiding any bias in their method of selection.
- The results should be presented clearly in a scientific way. The results should be understandable, numbers in tables should add up, and it should be obvious how any analyses were derived.
- The authors should describe how the quality of the papers was assessed – how many people assessed each paper, whether they were blinded to other researchers' opinions, what criteria of quality were used, whether these criteria were valid, reliable and reproducible, and whether they adhered to the criteria.
- The results should be relevant to the declared aim of the review.
- The results should be generalisable – the significance of different biases should be considered and their implications discussed. The author(s) should give a critical analysis of the scientific rigour of the studies in the review, with all interpretative remarks being justified.
- The results should be comprehensive. Negative as well as positive findings in the different studies should be described. The range of confidence limits gives more information than a mere probability statistic.
- The conclusions should be based on an overview of the data and/or analyses of all the studies included in the review.
- The outcomes should indicate clearly any modifications that should be made to future healthcare practice based on the evidence presented in the review.

If you want to practise your critical appraisal skills obtain a copy of the following review:

- Waddell G, Feder G, Lewis M. Systematic reviews of bed rest and advice to stay active for acute low back pain. *Br J Gen Pract* 1997; **47**: 647–52.

Read through the article first to get a feel for it. Then read it again conscientiously, absorbing the details and making notes as ideas and concerns come to mind. Now use the information given above, writing down your answers. The whole critical appraisal exercise should take you about three hours. Turn over and read how *we* reviewed this journal paper.

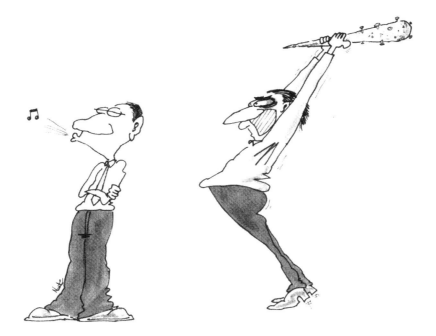

**It may be hard to convince your colleagues even when
you've got the evidence.**

Our review of Waddell G, Feder G, Lewis M. Systematic reviews of bed rest and advice to stay active for acute low back pain. *Br J Gen Pract* 1997; 47: 647–52.

This published review was prepared for the national *Guidelines on Acute Low Back Pain*,[39] an important and relevant problem in primary care. The following critique reflects the views of the authors and colleagues who attended the clinical effectiveness workshops. It is difficult to dissociate fact and interpretation in the critical appraisal of published papers and as several of the comments are matters of interpretation and opinion, you may well disagree with our critique.

Are the topic and purpose of the review clearly specified?

Yes. The aim was to review all randomised controlled trials of *bed rest* and of *advice to stay active* for acute back pain.

Were the search methods used comprehensive?

The search strategy was clearly stated and included searching Medline, EMBASE, hand searching and tracking down 'grey' materials. However, search of CINAHL was not included, which would have extended the search to include relevant literature from nursing and allied health professions such as occupational therapy and physiotherapy.

Did the review address a clearly focused issue?

No. The inclusion criteria were too vague. For example, one of the inclusion criteria stipulated 'back pain of up to three months' duration', but in some papers included in the review, the patients had had back pain for a few days, in others they had had pain for months. The inclusion criteria stated that trials of advice had to be set in 'primary care'. However, a very broad definition of primary care was used, e.g. three papers were set in occupational health clinics and emergency rooms.

The subjects in the bed rest studies and the advice populations were very different in regard to the settings, length of follow-up and different outcome measures (most of which were irrelevant according to Table 3) and, on the whole, smaller samples were used in the *bed rest* papers than in those about trials of *advice*.

Some papers concerned primary care, while others concerned hospital outpatient care. They included studies of patients with recurrent attacks, acute exacerbation of chronic back pain and sciatica. These are all groups of patients for whom optimum care may well be different and some may benefit from bed rest while other groups may not. They should have focused on a particular group or groups of patients, symptoms or settings.

There was no discussion of outcomes and the difficulties in measuring them. To sum up a paper as pain 'worse' or 'better' ignores the difficulties in assessing pain over a period of weeks. The most severe pain experienced or the duration of pain above a certain level, the average pain score, pain at rest or pain on activity are all important features.

Did the authors look for the appropriate papers to include in the review?

No. They should have been more focused. For example, they could have identified a clinical question such as 'Should patients with acute onset back pain be advised to rest in bed until the pain subsides, or should they be encouraged to stay active?' Then they should have searched for papers that reported trials comparing these two alternatives. Instead they treated *bed rest* and *advice* to stay active as separate interventions and carried out two separate reviews.

   Although the authors noted the problems with two of the papers and discussed them separately, they still included them in their review. For example, the paper by Pal *et al.* (1986) compared bed rest and continuous traction with bed rest and sham traction, which is a trial of traction and not a trial of bed rest at all. These papers should have been excluded.

   The authors state in the method that back schools were excluded, however one of the papers reviewed (Linequist *et al.* 1984) is a trial of a back school.

Do you think the important, relevant papers were included?

No, papers on end-point evaluation have not been considered.

If the results of the review have been combined was it reasonable to do so?

No, the studies have too little in common.

Did the authors do enough to assess the quality of the included studies?

No. There were too many dubious features of the scoring method used. The weighting of the criteria used for methodological scoring seems to have been accepted uncritically by the authors since it had been used in two other systematic reviews of back pain management. For example, an intention-to-treat analysis is one of the items (N) included in the methodological scoring system in Table 2. This is an essential feature, as a study loses nearly all of its credibility if it lacks this, and not just 5 points out of 100 as in the scoring system used by Waddell *et al*. 'Placebo controlled' is another one of the items (J) in the methodological scoring system. However, it is difficult to see how trials of bed rest and advice to stay active can be scored as to whether they are placebo controlled and how placebo bed rest might be arranged. A further problem with the methodological scoring is that the total sum in Table 2 is 100, yet the weightings given only add up to 95.

There is no substantive reason why co-interventions such as appropriate analgesia should be avoided in a study of back pain. To be realistic a trial protocol should allow appropriate analgesia, but should endeavour to ensure that patients in both groups are managed using the same guidelines with respect to analgesia. Use of analgesia could be an appropriate end-point to study.

What is the overall result of the review?

It is unclear because of the numerous flaws. The diversity of the studies in this area suggests that a more traditional type of review might be better, where papers are grouped under headings.

How precise are the results?

They only give results as 'better' or 'worse'. More precision is needed.

There are also several major mistakes. There is an inconsistency between Tables 2 and 3 in the total sum possible for the methodological scoring item F, which is given as 12 in Table 2 and 17 in Table 3. This accounts for the total adding up to 95 and not 100 as stated.

In Table 4 the asterisks and crosses in the last two entries appear to be mixed up. The asterisks should be crosses and the crosses should not be there.

Under *Methodological Quality*, the Spearman's rank correlation coefficient of 0.72 should not be interpreted as showing the rankings were similar – a value of 0.9 would be required.

The reporting of the results seems biased. In Tables 4 and 5 there are several instances where results are given as 'NS' (not significant) and several where the NS is elaborated on as 'slower recovery NS'. Where there is elaboration on NS, the detail, for example 'slower recovery (NS)', favours the final conclusion of the review. There must have been information available about all the 'NS' results and so the authors seem to have been selective in how much detail they present in order to favour their final conclusions.

Can the results be applied and generalised?

No, there are too many flaws. Furthermore, many of the studies included were not in primary care.

Were all important outcomes considered?

No, there is too little detail about outcomes, such as pain. Few of the important outcomes, such as time off work, were considered in the bed rest arm of the review.

Are the benefits worth the harms and costs?

This is unclear, given the flaws outlined above.

Stage 5

Apply the evidence

You have identified your problem, posed your question with help from colleagues at work, searched for the best available evidence, judged the quality of the evidence, weighed the relative importance of any conflicting results, applied the evidence theoretically to your own circumstances and situation, and now you should be ready to apply the evidence in practice.

Clinicians have expressed concern about the dangers of adhering blindly to evidence in practice, and fears that evidence-based practice might be regarded as the be-all and end-all as far as decisions about the cost-effective delivery of health services go. Clinical judgement and common sense must be paramount in keeping evidence in perspective. The information forming the 'evidence' may be irrelevant, incomplete or inaccurate, or the 'evidence' may simply not be applicable in the particular clinical circumstances in question. The NHS has a long way to go in accumulating a bank of good and reliable information about current clinical care and best practices.

Do not regard the evidence generated in randomised controlled trials as sacrosanct. They may provide the best sort of evidence for evaluating the benefits of alternative medications, but they are not necessarily the best way of identifying evidence for resolving more complex human health issues.

Evidence-based management has an even weaker information base than evidence-based clinical practice. It must be right to encourage practice managers and other health service managers to adopt a research culture with a questioning approach. This will encourage them to reflect about what is happening, how and why, and to compare management practices.

So bear all this in mind as you think about applying the evidence you have gained from your search to your particular clinical situation. You may like to think of making changes from the perspective of an individual clinician, a practice or unit, or a primary care organisation or hospital trust.

Diary of your progress in searching for evidence

Complete this summary of progress to date and your action plan for how you propose to introduce any changes in your working practices.

Write a summary of:

1 your problem (be as specific as possible so that you can measure the outcomes of any changes against this baseline position):

2 your question:

3 your search method – where you searched (databases, people):

4 the types of your best evidence (systematic review, randomised controlled trials, controlled trials, reports, conference proceedings, expert opinions):

5 ... give three titles of the most relevant and appropriate publications or sources that you found:

6 your conclusion(s) from the best evidence available in answer to your question:

7 the change(s) that you propose to make yourself or that others should make, as a result of the evidence you have obtained and the conclusion(s) you have drawn:

Action plan

People to whom you have fed back the results of the evidence:

Have you already written a timetabled action plan?   *Yes/No*

The baseline position:

Whom have you involved in discussions about the change(s) you propose?

Change(s) proposed:

People whom the proposed change(s) will affect:

Additional resources that will be required (people, premises, time, money, skills, etc.):

The timetable is:

Who will do what:

Advantages or health gains expected:

Disadvantages or losses (opportunity costs) that may happen:

How and when the changed situation will be monitored again:

Barriers to change

Once evidence has been gathered, projects have been completed and necessary changes discussed, there can still be many barriers to overcome before worthwhile changes can happen.

The King's Fund PACE[6] initiative identified the following barriers to change:

- others' lack of perception of the relevance of your proposed change (you should have realised this during your initial consultations with colleagues before you began)
- lack of resources to implement the change (time, staff, skills, equipment)
- short-term outlook of work colleagues
- conflicting priorities – without additional resources, changes have the potential to cause work overload or opportunity costs
- difficulties in measuring outcomes – it is difficult to find acceptable worthwhile health outcomes that are easily measured
- lack of necessary skills (forward planning is needed)
- no tradition of multidisciplinary working (this problem can probably only be surmounted with a culture change)
- limitations of research evidence on effectiveness (there is a lot more research about problems than there is about effective solutions)
- perverse incentives (a common flaw in the way the NHS functions)
- the intensity of others' contribution that is required (again consult early, get everyone on board and encourage everyone to 'own' your project).

And so ...

- anticipate the strength of evidence you will need to convince your colleagues that the efforts and costs of change will be worthwhile – to them and the patients. Do this through clinical governance – understand how to make clinical governance work for you in the next chapter.

Read more about the lessons to be learned in how to make successful changes happen.[6]

Stage 6

What clinical governance means and how to put it into practice

Clinical governance is inclusive, making quality everyone's business, whether they are a doctor or a nurse, manager or member of the administrative staff, a patient or a strategic planner. We need to know where we are now and where we want to get to if we are to drive up standards of healthcare. Clinical effectiveness and clinical audit are central to this process.[40]

'Clinical governance is the framework through which organisations influence the informal psychology and social functioning of their staff. Its delivery will result in every clinical team putting quality at the heart of their moment to moment care of patients. ... Clinical governance ... enables the vocation and motivation of healthcare professionals and patients by giving their personal energy a voice: allowing them to meaningfully and continuously improve the culture they are part of. It encapsulates an organisation's statutory responsibility for the delivery of safe, high quality patient care and it is the vehicle through which that accountable performance is made explicit.'[41]

Components of clinical governance

The components of clinical governance are well established. Bringing them together under the banner of clinical governance with explicit accountability for performance maintains quality in healthcare. The reception given to clinical governance ranges from an enthusiastic welcome to the cautious warning that innovations that improve quality may increase rather than decrease costs. Carefully evaluating your work and demonstrating subsequent improvements in patient care will enable you to form your own view about the place of clinical governance.

The following 14 themes are core components of professional and service development which, taken together, form a comprehensive approach to providing high-quality healthcare services and clinical governance. These are illustrated in the tree diagram:[40]

If you interweave these into your individual and workplace-based personal and professional development plans, you will have addressed the requirements for clinical governance at the same time.[42]

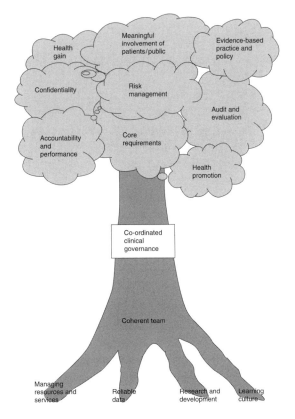

Figure 1:   'Routes' and branches of clinical governance (©2000 Chambers and Wakley).

1 **Learning culture**: in the practice, the primary care organisation, the trust and the NHS at large.
2 **Research and development culture**: throughout the health service.
3 **Reliable and accurate data**: in the practice, the primary care organisation and the NHS as a seamless whole.
4 **Well-managed resources and services**: as individuals, as a practice, as a primary care organisation or trust, across the NHS and in conjunction with social care and local authorities.
5 **Coherent team**: well-integrated teams within a practice, across a practice, in the primary care organisation or trust.
6 **Meaningful involvement of patients and the public**: in a practice or the NHS as a whole, including users, carers and the general population.

7 **Health gains**: activities to improve the health of patients in a practice, between practices, in the primary care organisation (PCO) or trust, and different geographical areas of the NHS.
8 **Confidentiality**: of information in consultations, in medical notes, between practitioners.
9 **Evidence-based practice and policy**: applying it in practice, in the primary care organisation or trust, in the district, across the NHS.
10 **Accountability and performance**: for standards, performance of individuals, the practice, primary care organisation or trust, health authority/board and the NHS, to the public and those in authority.
11 **Core requirements**: good fit with skill mix and whether individuals are competent to do their jobs, communication, workforce numbers, morale at practice level, across the NHS.
12 **Health promotion**: for patients, the public, opportunistic and in general, targeting those with most needs.
13 **Audit and evaluation**: for instance, of changes, of individuals' and practices' performance, of the primary care organisation's or trust's achievements, of district services.
14 **Risk management**: pro-active review, follow-up, risk management, risk reduction.

The challenges to delivering clinical governance

Delivering high-quality healthcare with guaranteed minimum standards of care for users at all times, is a major challenge. At present the quality of healthcare is patchy and variable. We aren't very good at detecting under-performance and then taking the initiative and rectifying it at an early stage. The small number of clinicians who do underperform exert a disproportionately large effect on the public's confidence. Causes of underperformance in an individual might relate to a lack of knowledge or skills, poor attitudes or ill health. A lack of management capability is nearly always an important contributory factor to inadequate clinical services or the provision of healthcare.

We need to understand why variation exists and explore ways of reducing inequalities. Variation in the quality of healthcare provided is common – between different practices in the same locality, between staff of the same discipline working in the same practice or unit, between care given to some groups of the population rather than others. There may be up to four-fold differences in rates of referral to hospital for a particular condition, between one doctor and another, for example; some practices have attached social workers and community psychiatric nurses while others do not, for instance.

Good practice means understanding and managing risk – both clinical and organisational aspects. Integrating risk management into all that you do is one of the key steps in preserving patient safety.[43] Identifying new cases of important conditions such as diabetes and undertaking audit more systematically will reduce the risks of omission – in detection and clinical management. The common areas of risk in providing healthcare services are:

- out-of-date clinical practice – and insufficient investment in staff learning
- lack of continuity of care
- poor communication – in the organisation, between clinician and patient
- mistakes in patient care – known and unknown
- patient complaints and lack of response to complaints
- financial risk – insufficient resources
- concerns about reputation – of organisation or individuals
- low staff morale.

Clinical governance offers a co-ordinated approach to overcoming these areas of risk through a blend of clinical and organisational improvements to the quality of healthcare practice. Initiatives such as practice-based commissioning present risks for both PCOs and practices. It adds complexity and requires sound governance and accountability.[44]

We need to agree on indicators of performance that are acceptable to clinicians and managers alike. It is often said that we tend to use outcomes that are the easiest to measure but which mean least in terms of the real quality of patient care.

Enhancing your personal and professional development

Education and training programmes should be relevant to service needs, whether at organisational or individual levels. Continuing professional development (CPD) programmes need to meet both the learning needs of individual health professionals and the wider service development needs of the NHS. You should no longer opt for CPD activities according to what you *want* to do, but rather, what you *need* to do. Clinical governance underpins professional and service development.[42]

Lifelong learning and CPD are integral to the concept of clinical governance and that includes everyone in a practice or department of a trust working towards agreed learning goals that are relevant to service development.

Practitioners can review the balance between their own and NHS priorities at their annual appraisal.

---

individual personal development plans
will feed into a
workplace- or practice-based personal and professional development plan
that will feed into
the organisation's business plan
all
underpinned by clinical governance[42]

Good morale and job satisfaction are prerequisites of learning and effective working, and should be nurtured by targeted personal and professional development plans. Clinical governance should be creating a culture and working environment where people thrive and feel fulfilled by their work.

The Royal College of General Practitioners has developed a variety of awards that recognise the high standards of quality of care achieved by a practitioner or a practice team – Fellowship by Assessment, Quality Practice Award, Quality Team Development and others. These require sustained CPD coupled with demonstrable high standards of care – clinical governance principles are integral to the process. The principles that underlie the Quality Team Development process are:[45]

- the criteria for assessment reflect the needs of patients
- professional self-regulation is the most effective and acceptable method of maintaining good professional practice
- the ethos should be educational, developmental and supportive
- every member of the primary healthcare team can take part
- the focus is the team, its functioning and the services it provides
- assessment should be multidisciplinary
- there should be local ownership and delivery.

1 How evidence-based care, clinical effectiveness and other components of clinical governance fit together: the practitioner's, the practice's or the unit's perspective[40]

Learning culture

You cannot learn about the cultural changes needed for providing multidisciplinary, team-based healthcare in the modern health service by sitting passively in a lecture. You need to experience the learning and interact with others who will be part of that new culture. Historically, health professionals have been keener to attend lectures than interactive educational activities such as organised small group sessions or informal teaching in their workplaces.

> The type or mode of education and training should be relevant to the topic of the learning and the characteristics or circumstances of the 'students'.

Maximising learning about the new requirements of the NHS will involve:

- setting up in-house formal and informal education and training opportunities
- everyone creating personal development plans that incorporate all modes of learning: reading and reflecting, shadowing others, small group discussions, online materials, as well as lectures and seminars
- a practice- or directorate-wide approach to a topic so that a portfolio of experience is built up to which everyone contributes – useful for revalidation and re-registration of team members' professional qualifications.

> Using a questionnaire is full of pitfalls and it is one of the most difficult techniques for gaining a true or valid answer to the question posed.

Applying research and development in practice

One of the most common research and development activities undertaken by health professionals is a questionnaire survey of their patients. A poorly designed patient satisfaction survey will give you meaningless results so that all the time and effort spent on the satisfaction survey is wasted, and changes made as a result of such a survey still do not satisfy the patient population. Patient satisfaction questionnaires are commonly used in hospital and general practice, as a hybrid of research and audit. Novices may mistakenly believe that undertaking a questionnaire survey is one of the simplest and easiest methods.

To try and ensure that a patient satisfaction survey is a meaningful exercise:

- use a questionnaire that has been tried and tested by someone else and is valid for your workplace setting
- make sure that the questions are relevant and appropriate to the purpose of the enquiry
- use questions which have an easily answered format with simple choices of response
- use appropriate language likely to be understood by all respondents, with translations into other languages if there are non-English speakers in your target population
- avoid leading questions that imply you are expecting a particular answer, otherwise respondents will tend to give the answer implied as being the 'right' one because they want to please you
- pilot your draft questionnaire to detect problems with your questions or method.

Reliable and accurate data

Clinicians, patients and administrators need reliable and accurate data to connect individuals or their healthcare records to other knowledge that is relevant to the care of the patient.

Set standards for a general practice:

- summarise medical records; within a specified time period for records of new patients
- review dates for checks on medication; with audit in place to monitor standards adhered to and plan for underperformance if necessary
- establish chronic disease registers and keep them updated
- use computers for diagnostic recording

- record information from external sources – hospital, other organisations – relevant to individual patients or the practice as a whole.

Think of the data you should collect about your or others' performance too. There should be 'effective systems in place to give early warning of any failure or potential failure in clinical performance ....'[46]

Well-managed resources and services

The things you need to achieve best practice should be in the right place at the right time and working correctly every time.
  Set standards in your workplace for:

- access to premises and availability of services for people with special needs, such as those with sensory and visual impairments
- provision of routine and urgent appointments
- access to and provision for referral for investigation or treatment
- pro-active monitoring of chronic illness and disability
- alternatives to face-to-face consultations
- consultation length.

The six primary care services to which the public requires access are: information, advice, triage and treatment, continuity of care, personal care and other services.[47] Minimising inequalities and the outcomes of new skill-mix models are two prime concerns at the heart of considerations about access and evaluating standards, especially with regard to:

- level of access versus quality of care received
- access for those who demand more versus equity of access for all based on need
- an impersonal service versus continuity of care versus personal care
- a demand-led (by patients) service versus a service that is prioritised or rationed
- access to one particular member of the care team, first or above others
- substitution of, or delegation to, staff members.

Systems should be designed to prevent and detect errors. So keep systems simple and sensible, and inform everyone how systems operate so that they are less likely to bypass the system or make errors.
  Concentrate on ensuring that your systems are designed to deliver care that is:

- safe
- effective
- accessible
- reliable

- efficient
- timely
- equitable
- patient-centred.[48]

Coherent teamwork

Teams produce better patient care than single practitioners operating in a fragmented way. Effective teams make the most of the different contributions of individual clinical disciplines in delivering patient care. The characteristics of effective teams are:

- shared ownership of a common purpose
- clear goals for the contributions each discipline makes
- open communication between team members
- opportunities offered for team members to enhance their skills.

A team approach helps different team members adopt an evidence-based approach to patient care, by having to justify their approach to the rest of the team.[49]

The experiences of teamwork on the Wirral[49]

The team was composed by a family support worker employed by the voluntary sector joining a community psychiatric nursing team. They found that the factors that helped the team to work well were:

- that each member of the team had a separate function
- joint training which cemented the team, although obstacles from different employer arrangements had to be overcome
- interdisciplinary differences of opinion about patient care being welcomed as a way of increasing debate and generating a wider range of options for care.

Meaningful involvement of patients and the public

The terms 'user' and 'public' are employed here to include patients or users, carers, non-users of services, the local community, a particular subgroup of the population and the general public.

If user involvement and public participation are done well they should result in:

- reductions in health inequalities

- better outcomes of individual care
- better health for the population
- better quality and more locally responsive services
- greater ownership of health services
- a better understanding of why and how local services need to be changed and developed.

Public participation may be organised at five levels and you should aim for true participation at the fifth level whenever possible:[50]

- **Level 1**: information exchange
- **Level 2**: consultation: the public and patients express their views but the consultant makes the decisions
- **Level 3**: support: the public decides what to do and others support them in doing it
- **Level 4**: deciding together: thinking and planning together
- **Level 5**: acting together: putting plans into action together.

A meaningful public consultation involves the exchange of information between the healthcare providers and the general public, obtaining a representative opinion as a result that feeds into the local decision-making process of healthcare services or whoever is sponsoring the consultation.

How to go about undertaking meaningful consultation[51]

Be clear about:

- the purpose of the exercise: is it important and is it necessary?
- the type and identity of the population to whom the purpose relates
- how to reach and engage the target population
- the extent and mode of information exchange required prior to consultation
- the implications of the methods you employ in the consultation – what outputs you expect from the consultation
- how you will act on the results of the consultation
- how you will feed back the outcome of the consultation exercise
- how you will evaluate the consultation exercise.

You may have to trade off a relatively cheaper method of consultation that engages with fewer people or with a less representative section of the population subgroup; if you do, you will need to understand what biases are arising and make allowances for those biases when you interpret the results of the consultation.

Health gains

Take the example of coronary heart disease (CHD).

Modifiable risk factors for CHD include: cigarette smoking, raised blood pressure, body composition, lack of physical exercise, total serum cholesterol and excessive alcohol consumption.

Maximising the reduction in patients' risk factors for CHD in general practice, for example, will involve:

- identifying patients who will benefit from medical interventions, e.g. you might identify patients for secondary prevention of ischaemic heart disease by extracting information from repeat prescriptions for nitrates and/or aspirin, looking through medical records for patients with specific conditions (e.g. post-myocardial infarction, angina) or who have been classified as having CHD and entered on the practice computer
- targeting those patients once identified in systematic ways and auditing the results of your campaign
- discussing CHD risks as a practice team so that everyone has a similar understanding of the risks and benefits, gives out consistent messages and recommends similar interventions
- using the most up-to-date interventions with best outcomes, e.g. in your approach to smoking cessation
- remembering that a patient's perceived risk or susceptibility is an important determinant of whether the patient takes preventive action.

Confidentiality

Confidentiality is a component of clinical governance that may be overlooked. Experienced health professionals and managers may assume that junior or new staff know all about confidentiality, but, of course, they may not. There are many tricky situations where one person asks for information about another's clinical condition – test results or a progress report – where it is not clear-cut as to whether this information should be supplied or withheld, or even if the person asked should acknowledge that the person enquired about is under their care. If the person in question is terminally ill and within a few days of death, the health professional will want to prepare the relatives; if the person with the terminal illness is functioning well, then their medical attendants will not be able to share medical information without the patient's express permission.

The Caldicott committee report[52] describes principles of good practice to safeguard confidentiality when information is being used for non-clinical purposes:

- justify the purpose
- do not use patient-identifiable information unless it is absolutely necessary
- use the minimum necessary patient-identifiable information
- access to patient-identifiable information should be on a strict need-to-know basis
- everyone with access to patient-identifiable information should be aware of his or her responsibilities.

Evidence-based culture: policy and practice

The key features of whether or not local guidelines worked in one initiative were that:[53]

- there was multidisciplinary involvement in drawing them up
- a well-described systematic review of the literature underpinned the guidelines with graded recommendations for best practice linked to the evidence
- ownership was nurtured at a national and local level
- a local implementation plan ensured that all the practicalities (time, staff, education and training, resources) were foreseen and met, stakeholders were supported, predictors of sustainability addressed – guideline usability, individualising guidelines to practitioners and patients.

Clinicians may rebel against new policies that they perceive as being out of line with patients' needs, and policy makers may become frustrated at the intransigence of those in practice – if there is a gulf between those driving policy and those responsible for practice. The evidence base justifying health policy and management decisions in relation to a particular service is just as important as the evidence base for the clinical care component of the service or the education of staff providing that service.

Incorporating research-based evidence into everyday practice should promote policies on effective working and improve quality and a clinical governance culture.

- Be sure of the evidence for a proposed policy and the best way to implement it. Search for the evidence or set up a formal evaluation where there is insufficient evidence for the best way.
- Consult widely and early when any policy decision is being made, demonstrating how the input to that consultation was incorporated into the final policy.
- Base management and policy decisions on accurate information.
- Negotiate necessary changes in the organisation and management of the practice and carefully cascade information about the changes throughout the practice team or organisation.
- Provide adequate resources to underpin strategies to change practice, such as people to promote that change who have the right levels of knowledge and skills.
- Incorporate monitoring and evaluation of the change from the planning stage and throughout the activity.
- Find ways to maintain and reinforce the new practices, e.g. reminder systems, educational outreach programmes.
- Disseminate information about the change in ways that are appropriate to the nature and setting of the participants.

Accountability and performance

Health professionals – particularly GPs, pharmacists and dentists with their self-employed status – do not always realise that they are accountable to others from outside their own profession. But in fact they are accountable to:

- the general public – who are entitled to expect high standards of healthcare
- the profession – to maintain standards of knowledge and skills of the profession as a whole
- the government and employers – who expect high standards of healthcare from the workforce.

> Health professionals who believe that they are not accountable to others may be reluctant to collect the evidence to demonstrate that they are fit to practise, and that their working environment is fit to practise from, the basis of the evidence for revalidation of their professional qualifications. In addition, they may not co-operate with central NHS standards such as those set out in the National Service Frameworks or in *Standards for Better Health*.[54]

Identify and rectify underperformance at an early stage by:[55]

- regular appraisals (at least annually) linked into clinical governance and personal development plans. Appraisal is a process of regular meetings between manager and staff member with support for the benefit of the member of staff
- detecting those who have significant health problems and referring them for help
- systematic audit that detects individuals' performance as opposed to the overall performance of the practice or unit's team
- an open learning culture where team members are discouraged from covering up colleagues' inadequacies so that problems can be resolved at an early stage.

Many of the misunderstandings that arise between patients and doctors have potential or actual adverse consequences. Fourteen categories of misunderstanding were identified in one study of prescribing relating to patient information unknown to the doctor, doctor information unknown to the patient, conflicting information, disagreement about attribution of side effects, failure of communication and relationship factors. This study demonstrated how dependent clinical management is on good organisational systems manned by non-clinical staff, and how important it is that patients participate in the consultation.[56]

Health promotion

People may underestimate relative risks as applied to themselves and their own behaviour, e.g. many smokers accept the relationship between smoking tobacco and disease, but do not believe that they are personally at risk. People usually have a reasonable idea of the relative risks of various activities and behaviours, although their personal estimates of the magnitude of risks tend to be biased – small probabilities are often overestimated and high probabilities are often underestimated.[57]

You need to understand the terms used to be able to extrapolate the messages from a research paper to explain the risks and benefits to others. You need critical appraisal skills to be able to form an opinion as to whether you can depend on the results from a research study. There are some publications where much of the work of interpreting results from research studies has been done for you in a reliable way (see www.ebandolier.com).[58]

Audit and evaluation

We should be looking for ways of assessing qualities like clinicians' and NHS managers' kindness, empathy, (clinical) reasoning and listening skills, as well as more tangible measures of the quality of care.

Analysis of critical incidents should focus on organisational factors as well as the performance of particular individuals.

Undertake regular audits of aspects of the structure, process and outcome of a service or development in your practice or department. See if you have achieved what you expected when you established the criteria and standards of the audit programme. Check out that you have completed the full cycle of the audit, including making changes and re-auditing.[59]

> 'When pathways and protocols are developed, an audit tool needs to be created to allow prospective evaluation of the care delivered and the outcomes achieved, including quality-of-life measures. Clinical teams and patients should be involved in determining how best to record outcomes, so that the measures developed address what really matters to patients.'[60]

Evaluation is essential to find out how well things are going. That could be checking out your experience in your post – such as the development of your knowledge and skills or how the team members work together, or how well you are delivering a service to patients. How else will you know if your efforts have been worthwhile, or if you could improve the way you do things? Incorporate evaluation into any plan to establish new staff posts, or where you vary what work staff do, right from the beginning. Keep your evaluation as simple as possible and avoid wasting resources on an unnecessarily bureaucratic type of evaluation.

Like all quality assurance processes, an evaluation should be:

- efficient, effective and economical – in relation to the costs and effectiveness of what you are evaluating as well as the evaluation process itself
- valid – evaluating what it is intended to measure
- reliable – producing consistent and accurate findings
- flexible and practical
- fair – not favouring any aspect; being inclusive
- in proportion – to the specific issues being evaluated
- accountable –specify lines of responsibility
- co-ordinated – with other development or review processes.[59]

Core requirements

You cannot deliver clinical governance without well-trained and competent staff, the right skill-mix of staff and a safe and comfortable working environment, all providing cost-effective care.

Following published referral guidelines may increase healthcare costs, which should be justifiable as cost-effective care when all direct and indirect costs are taken into account.

Your healthcare team can do much under the umbrella of clinical governance to respond to the national challenges to improve:

- partnership: working together across the NHS to ensure the best possible care
- performance: acting to review and deliver higher standards of healthcare
- the professions and wider workforce: breaking down barriers between different disciplines
- patient care: access, convenient services, empowerment to take a full part in decision making about their own medical care and in planning and providing health services in general
- prevention: promoting healthy living across all sections of society and tackling variations in care.

Risk management

Risk management in general practice or a trust mainly centres on 'facts' rather than 'values' or 'preferences'. These are the facts about what the probability is that a hazard will give rise to harm – how bad is the risk, how likely is the risk, when will the risk happen, if ever, and how certain are we of our estimates about the risk? This applies just as much whether the risk is an environmental or organisational risk in the practice, or a clinical risk.[61]

Communicating and managing risks with individual patients is very much about finding ways to explain risks and elicit people's values and preferences, so that all these dimensions can be incorporated into the decisions they make themselves to take risks or choose between alternatives that involve different risks and benefits.[62] A well-functioning system through which patients can make complaints and receive feedback on the outcome should allow the practice or unit to reduce the risk of a recurrence.

Travel health, for instance, is an example of risk management that requires consideration of clinical and organisational risks, which are minimised or eliminated.

> *The risks* of acquiring infections from travelling abroad are greater if people are not aware of the specific risks of disease and do not take appropriate precautions.

Risk management to reduce the chances of a traveller contracting an avoidable disease from abroad involves:

- having a consistent policy in your practice team for advice given for types of vaccination for specific countries and situations
- being able to signpost patients to travel advice centres and sources of information for further help, e.g. yellow fever centre and Internet sites
- encouraging patients to complete their courses of immunisation after they have returned from holiday to give them longer-lasting immunity
- good stock control of immunisations stored in the surgery, so you do not have an excessive quantity which then exceeds its 'best before' date and you do not run out of stocks and disappoint patients.

> Chemoprophylaxis to avoid malaria is only one part of a preventive approach – awareness of the risk by traveller and doctor, reducing bites from mosquitoes, and awareness of the residual risk with prompt diagnosis and treatment of clinical malaria are all components of risk management.

2 How evidence-based care, clinical effectiveness and other components of clinical governance fit together: the primary care organisation's or trust's perspective[40]

The 14 components of clinical governance described apply just as much to the approach required by a primary care organisation or trust as they do to practices and individual health professionals. But they must also set up:

- clear lines of responsibility and accountability for the overall quality of clinical care across their organisation for the area covered by their patient population

- a systematic approach to monitoring and developing clinical standards in practices
- a comprehensive programme of quality improvement systems including workforce planning and development
- education and training plans
- clear policies aimed at managing risk
- integrated procedures for all professional groups to identify and remedy poor performance
- a culture where education, research and sharing good practice are valued.

Clinical governance will be part of a culture of learning and the organisation will have an ethos of participation – for staff and patients to engage in quality improvement.

The Healthcare Commission and its predecessors work with trusts in England (with some duties in Wales) to improve quality through monitoring and service development.

It covers primary care trusts (PCTs), hospital and specialist trusts, ambulance trusts, mental health trusts, care trusts and learning disability trusts. It does not include non-NHS organisations. The aim is to make sure that NHS trusts reach basic standards of healthcare and to encourage them to do better in future.

The annual health check is the Healthcare Commission's way of finding out how well NHS trusts are performing.[63] It checks how far they are meeting the Government's *Standards for Better Health*.[54]

Trusts receive a score of excellent, good, fair or weak for their standards of quality and use of resources, replacing the previous system of awarding a single 'star rating' to trusts. The quality element is derived from all of the components of the annual health check, except for use of resources. The quality of services is reviewed from a clinical point of view looking at how patients and the public actually experience them. The quality of care score covers core standards, existing targets, new national targets and the outcomes of improvement reviews and acute hospital portfolio studies. The use of resources element is based on an assessment of how effectively an organisation manages its financial resources.

The four high level questions at the core of the annual health check are:

- is care safe and clinically effective?
- are services accessible and patient focused?
- is public money used efficiently and effectively?
- is action being taken to improve and protect the health of local people and tackle inequalities?

To demonstrate good clinical governance, the primary care organisation or trust should be able to show that:

- users and carers believe that they are well cared for
- all staff feel included, listened to, and empowered in their roles
- all staff understand and own clinical governance
- there is an integrated strategy for the implementation of clinical governance
- the board has patient safety and service quality at the top of its agenda
- they identify and act on the areas of most concern to the organisation
- there is clear evidence of significant improvement in organisational performance.[64]

Action plan for the next 12 months for XXXX Primary Care Organisation – an example

1 Establish and organise clinical governance infrastructure:

- support practices' clinical governance leads: cascade to leads in all practices and other organisations in the constituency
- organise the gathering of reliable data: efficient input and retrieval of data, prioritising data
- provide protected time in practice for: building up infrastructure, undertaking quality improvement and support
- keep trust's requirements of practices simple in short term: aim for co-operation rather than verification of their performance, for now
- help practices understand what is required of them: linked to data that primary care organisation must collect for the Healthcare Commission and other inspection agencies
- demonstrate benefits of clinical governance, e.g. by compiling example portfolios of evidence for revalidation of professional qualifications, disseminating real examples of good chronic disease management and better patient management
- infrastructure in practices will be individualised according to practice characteristics and size.

2 Suggest clinical topics as example areas to build clinical governance infrastructure at practice (or unit) level, e.g. management of coronary heart disease (CHD):

- practice profile template: staffing, premises, facilities at the practice, recent audit activity, level of patient involvement and participation, special services offered or planned, professional development activities, how information technology is used, risk management approach
- clinical checklist of best practice: checklist around CHD theme will include standards and timetabled programmes for health promotion, lifestyle, family history, smoking, medication and standards for access for routine, semi-urgent,

---

emergency consultations (i.e. a mix of pro-active/reactive standards) evidence submitted for the Quality and Outcomes Framework
- gain consensus across the trust about what standards are acceptable
- establish baseline of what professionals currently do, to highlight gaps and duplication in relation to standards
- get feedback from patients about current services (via national survey, published literature and local consultation exercises)
- identify what works from the Cochrane Library
- summarise existing standards and protocols, looking at how they match with 'gold' standards given in the Cochrane Library, and the guidance from the National Institute for Health and Clinical Excellence (NICE)
- identify the skill base of staff across the trust's constituency in relation to CHD
- identify the core standards expected in primary care (for instance in the National Service Framework for CHD, the health improvement programme)
- feed back the above to practices and encourage them to identify their timed action plans to deliver clinical and infrastructure goals, what resources/ support they need (include checklist of what they could ask for) and who leads in the practice on that clinical topic, education and training, clinical governance and other priority areas.

3 Areas in which the trust could offer practical support:

- staff training, focused on the Quality and Outcomes Framework
- advise on maintenance and application of disease registers and other common information systems
- shared use of specialist nurses
- IT training to understand best practice in recall systems; sharing expertise between highly developed practices and needy ones
- raising awareness about the meaning and implementation of clinical governance
- initial prioritisation of most needy practices from baseline assessment of performance
- disseminate information to practices – written material, seminars, workshops, personal contact, etc.
- scope of skill base across organisation – expertise of staff and good models of practice
- run educational sessions linking with continuing professional development tutors and multidisciplinary training. Feed in learning needs identified at annual appraisals. Trawl what is available and where there are gaps commission education – local workshops; link to scheduled training (receptionist, nurse training); arrange training about practice-based learning plans; training about skills in user involvement/public consultation; link to roadshows for patients and the public
- identify practice needs against defined standards, i.e. against agreed practice checklists of good practice considering infrastructure, clinical management of CHD
- patients' and public's views actively sought at trust level and disseminated to practices

- encourage innovations by demonstrating their significant benefits, based on evidence.

4 Evaluate activities:

- agree short-term and longer-term outcomes with individual and groups of practices; aim to reach surrogative targets as per agreed standards; measure achievement of improved care/services against standards.

Threats to a coherent clinical governance programme in your practice or unit are:

- lack of consensus and teamwork in practice or unit
- lack of understanding of priorities, or lack of overlap between the requirements of the Quality and Outcomes Framework or other organisational priorities and patients' needs
- staff thinking 'what's the point' if no resources for change?
- 'blame' culture – way of thinking
- geographic isolation of some staff and practices
- lack of trust and information about skills between health professions, or people's doubts about substitution involved in skill-mix
- suspicion of small practices that they will be criticised or have their priorities swamped by larger practices
- fear of new things/deficit in skills to cope with rapid change
- lack of time to fit new things in and get involved
- less well performing practices or units may find providing comparative data threatening
- clinical governance leads in primary care organisation or trust may be seen as 'know it alls' and 'do it alls' by other local practices, who then leave them to it
- practitioners being unsure how best to proceed to blend clinical governance in with continuing professional development
- lack of ownership of the importance of clinical governance by 'ordinary' practitioners
- clinical governance being seen as a threat and as a top-down imposition by some
- lack of multidisciplinary culture or ownership – not all members of the practice or workplace team see themselves with a part to play in clinical governance
- anxieties about how information on performance will be used and interpreted
- staff sickness levels may create variations in the delivery of services and blips of underperformance if there is no backfill

- lack of systematic staff training with good strategic leadership
- patient expectations may exceed the capacity to deliver
- staff turnover may be detrimental, e.g. loss of experience in applying disease registers and recall systems
- some small isolated practices or specialty units may find it hard to share information and resources with peers
- lack of opportunities/willingness to learn about clinical governance in some practices or units
- low level of patient or public involvement in practice or unit, so standards are set by healthcare staff rather than the public
- worries about identifying weaknesses within team or to employer or outside person which may become source of blame
- health professionals may not see the wider context of the contributions of non-health organisations to improving health, nor understand each others' roles or the potential of the services each offers.

A recent National Audit Office report[65] found that there were clear indications of changes to a culture supporting clinical governance and that individual components of clinical governance were mainly in place in most trusts. The range of achievements included:

- clinical quality issues being more mainstream
- structures and organisational arrangements to make clinical governance happen being in place
- clinical governance being well established and embedded in the corporate systems of virtually all trusts
- progress in the development of a more co-ordinated, coherent and consistent clinical governance strategy in trusts.

One hospital approach to clinical governance was to reform the senior committee structure to reflect:[66]

- leadership at different levels
- multidisciplinary style
- active co-ordination of the different elements of the committee, and of the hospital
- sharing of work across the service.

To achieve this, lead roles and responsibilities were allotted so that:

- evidence-based practice was led by a consultant psychiatrist
- risk management was led by a forensic psychologist
- a nurse manager led on policy and procedure
- the senior occupational therapist led on clinical audit
- a general manager led on user issues and complaints.

The Healthcare Concordat is a voluntary agreement between organisations that regulate, audit, inspect or review elements of health and healthcare in England. So, inspections are co-ordinated with other reviews and collections of data and focus on the experiences of patients, other users of services and carers. Inspections support improvements in quality and performance, and are targeted and proportionate. The website includes a range of tools, including a scheduling tool which allows signatory bodies to co-ordinate their visits to providers of healthcare.[67]

Full signatories to the Healthcare Concordat are the:

- Healthcare Commission
- Audit Commission
- National Audit Office
- Mental Health Act Commission
- Commission for Social Care Inspection
- Health and Safety Executive
- NHS Litigation Authority
- Academy of Medical Royal Colleges
- Post Graduate Medical Education and Training Board
- Conference of Postgraduate Deans
- General Medical Council
- Human Fertilisation and Embryology Authority
- NHS Counter Fraud and Security Management Service
- Skills for Health.

3 Research Governance Framework for Health and Social Care

Research is essential to health and wellbeing and to the development of modern and effective services. Just as clinical governance aims to continually improve the standards of clinical care and to reduce unacceptable variations in clinical practice, *research governance* aims to continually improve the standards of research and to reduce unacceptable variations in research practice. Research governance applies across health and social care and aims to enhance the partnership between health services and science.

The *Research Governance Framework for Health and Social Care*[68] defines the broad principles of good research governance and is the key to ensuring that health and social care research is conducted to high scientific and ethical standards. The Research Governance Framework spans the responsibilities of individuals and organisations involved in research, outlines delivery systems and standards to improve research quality and safeguard the public and describes local and national monitoring systems. It involves enhancing ethical and scientific quality, promoting good practice, reducing adverse incidents, ensuring lessons are learned and preventing poor performance and misconduct. The *Research Governance Framework for Health and Social Care* is summarised in the box below.

Research Governance Framework for Health and Social Care

What does research governance do?

- sets standards in research and defines the mechanisms to deliver those standards
- describes the monitoring and assessment arrangements
- improves research quality and safeguards the public by:
  - enhancing the ethical and scientific quality of research
  - promoting good practice in research
  - reducing adverse incidents in research and ensuring lessons are learned
  - preventing poor performance and misconduct in research.

Who is research governance for?

- managers and staff, in all professional groups, no matter how senior or junior and for all those who:
  - participate in research
  - host research in their organisation
  - fund research proposals or infrastructure
  - manage research
  - undertake research
- everyone working in all health and social care research environments, including:
  - primary care
  - secondary care
  - tertiary care
  - social care
  - public health.

What does research governance cover?

- ethics
- science
- information
- health, safety and employment
- finance and intellectual property.

Where can I get research governance documents?

- An updated edition of the *Research Governance Framework for Health and Social Care* for **England** is on the web at: www.dh.gov.uk

- The Scottish Executive *Research Governance Framework for Health and Community Care* is on the web at: www.show.scot.nhs.uk/CSO/ Publications/ResGov/Framework/RGFEdTwo.pdf
- The *Research Governance Framework for Health and Social Care* in **Wales** is being updated and may be accessed through www.dh.gov.uk
- The *Research Governance Framework for Health and Social Care* in **Northern Ireland** is at: www.dh.gov.uk/assetRoot/04/06/67/68/04066768. pdf

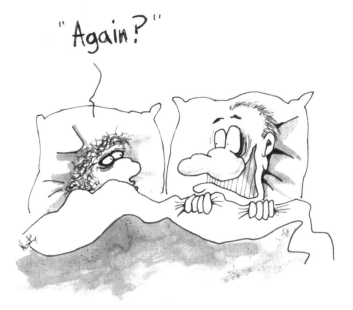

Once you've tried to apply clinical effectiveness – you'll want to do it again!

EVALUATE YOUR NEWLY GAINED KNOWLEDGE AND SKILLS IN CLINICAL EFFECTIVENESS AND CLINICAL GOVERNANCE

Evaluate how much you have learned by doing this programme and compare your answers to questions 1 and 2 below with the equivalent questions in your initial self-assessment of your knowledge and skills about the topic at the beginning of this book.

Please circle as many answers as apply or fill in the information requested.

1 How confident do you feel *now* that you know enough about clinical effectiveness to be able to:

Ask a relevant question?	*Very*	*Somewhat*	*Not at all*
Undertake a search of the literature?	*Very*	*Somewhat*	*Not at all*
Find readily available evidence?	*Very*	*Somewhat*	*Not at all*
Weigh up available evidence?	*Very*	*Somewhat*	*Not at all*
Decide if changes in practice are warranted?	*Very*	*Somewhat*	*Not at all*
Make changes in practice as appropriate?	*Very*	*Somewhat*	*Not at all*

2 Which database(s) have you used in this programme?

Medline   Cochrane   OMNI   Other (what?)

3 What level of evidence did you find in answer to your question (or main question if you posed more than one question)?

Strong evidence from at least one systematic review of multiple, well-designed randomised controlled trials (RCTs).

Strong evidence from at least one properly designed RCT of appropriate size.

Evidence from well-designed trials without randomisation.

Evidence from well-designed non-experimental studies from more than one centre or research group.

Opinions of well-respected authorities, based on clinical evidence, descriptive studies or reports of expert committees.

No evidence at all.

4 To whom have you given a report about the evidence you found?
   Colleagues at work   Friends/family   Bosses (managers) at work
   Other (who?)

5 What is/are the outcome(s) of you asking your main question and finding the evidence?

   Made change(s) to an aspect of work – if so, please describe what change(s) you have made or plan to make, who was involved in deciding to make the change(s), who is involved in the new change(s), whether you need any more resources or training and how you will review the change(s):

   Decided against making any change(s) to any aspect of work – if so, why did you decide not to make any change(s) and who was involved in that decision?

   Other outcome – what?

6 How will you use your new-found knowledge about clinical effectiveness in the future?

7 A practice nurse and therapist with whom you work have been given the task of triaging patients requesting emergency appointments. The nurse sees all the patients except for those complaining of musculoskeletal pain of some sort, who are referred to the physio at the next appointment. Lots of patients are complaining to you how difficult it is to see a doctor nowadays, the nurse and therapist moan because too little time has been allocated to see these extra patients and the additional training they've been promised has not materialised. What do you do? (Circle all that apply.)

   Nothing – it's not your responsibility.

   Inform the patients how to complain.

Log the patients' complaints and report them to the practice manager.

Encourage the nurse and therapist to take their concerns to the next practice team meeting.

Support the nurse and therapist in reviewing the operation of the new system with the practice manager and clinical governance lead.

(Hopefully, your own response will reflect the position that everyone working in the NHS is responsible for the quality of care their team provides.)

8 You have just been appointed as the clinical governance lead in your workplace. What are your roles and responsibilities likely to be and how will you go about promoting a positive culture of clinical governance among your team members?

Write down your answers – you can glean the information you need from Stage 6, which is the chapter on applying clinical governance in practice.

USEFUL PUBLICATIONS OF EVIDENCE ALREADY AVAILABLE

Some evidence is already available, so it is not necessary to appraise all the evidence yourself. The following resources will be useful.

Bandolier is a UK journal published by the Pain Relief Unit at Oxford which provides key evidence about the effectiveness of healthcare, reviewing national and international evidence. It is available by personal subscription. It is available in full text on the Internet at www.ebandolier.com

Clinical Evidence is a compendium of evidence on the effects of common clinical interventions, published by the BMJ Publishing Group. It is updated and expanded every six months and summarises the best available evidence about the prevention and treatment of a wide range of clinical conditions. A plus point is that its contents are driven by questions rather than by the availability of research evidence and so it identifies gaps in the evidence, leaving you to make your own decisions. *Clinical Evidence* is freely available to all, www.clinicalevidence.com/ceweb/conditions/index.jsp

Clinical Governance Bulletin is a quarterly publication from the Royal Society of Medicine Press to which institutions and individuals can subscribe. The contents report and review quality aspects of local initiatives in primary and secondary healthcare. The Bulletin has an emphasis on practical 'how we did it' material. It is distributed free to some NHS professionals with financial support from The Health Foundation. Full text is online at www.rsmpress. co.uk/cgb.htm

Drug & Therapeutics Bulletin (DTB) provides independent evaluations of drugs and other medical treatments and management issues. See www. dtb.org.uk/idtb/

In May 2006, the Department of Health withdrew the funding for free provision of DTB for the NHS. You may still have access via your Athens password: check with your healthcare library.

Evidence-Based Medicine provides critical appraisals of systematic reviews and primary research, with a commentary from a clinical expert. Much of the journal content is available as part of the Evidence Based Medicine Reviews (EBMR) database by subscription from OVID at www.ovid.com/site/catalog/

Database/904.jsp?top=2&mid=3&bottom=7&subsection=10 Print subscriptions are available from the BMJ Publishing Group, BMA House, Tavistock Square, London WC1H 9JR. See www.ebm. bmjjournals.com

HSTAT(Health Services/Technology Assessment Text) Clinical guidelines from the US Agency for Healthcare Research and Quality. Full text guidelines and summaries of the systematic reviews on which they are based. See www.ncbi.nlm.nih.gov/books/bv.fcgi?rid=hstat

MeReC Bulletin is aimed at GPs and pharmacists and provides reviews of new drugs, covering issues of safety, effectiveness, cost, appropriateness and acceptability. It is available online at www.npc.co.uk/merec_index.htm

Netting the Evidence provides an evidence-based virtual library and is the closest thing on the Web to a 'one-stop shop' for evidence-based healthcare. See www.shef.ac.uk/scharr/ir/netting

Organisations

Aggressive Research Intelligence Facility (ARIF)
ARIF is a specialist unit funded by the NHS Executive, West Midlands. The role of the unit is to improve the incorporation of research findings into population-level healthcare decisions in the NHS by helping healthcare workers access and interpret research evidence, particularly systematic reviews of research. Although ARIF has a regional role, it will attempt to help all callers. The website provides summaries of the research information ARIF has uncovered in response to requests received. The website is at: www.arif.bham.ac.uk

Centre for Reviews and Dissemination (CRD)
CRD is a sibling organisation of the UK Cochrane Centre, funded by the Department of Health to provide information on the effectiveness and cost-effectiveness of treatments and the delivery and organisation of healthcare. CRD carries out systematic reviews, provides a database of good quality reviews, offers a dissemination and information service and helps to promote research-based practice in the NHS. CRD plays an important role in disseminating the contents of Cochrane reviews to NHS decision makers. It provides an information and enquiry service on reviews and economic evaluations for healthcare professionals, purchasers and providers, NHS managers, information providers, health service researchers and consumer organisations. Its main outputs are: Database of Abstracts of Reviews of Effects (DARE); NHS Economic Evaluation Database (NHSEED); and the Health Technology Assessment (HTA) Database. Centre for Reviews and Dissemination, University of

York, York YO1 5DD. Tel: 01904 433707. Email: crd@york.ac.uk The website is at: www.york.ac.uk/inst/crd/

National Institute for Health and Clinical Excellence (NICE)
NICE provides NHS patients, health professionals and the public in England and Wales with authoritative, robust and reliable guidance on current 'best practice'. This is regularly updated and offers guidance on appraisals of new and existing health technologies, the clinical management of specific conditions and clinical audit. Information about the Institute and its work is available on their website at: www.nice.org.uk

Useful websites include:

- CASP (Critical Appraisal Skills Programme):
  www.phru.nhs.uk/casp/casp.htm
- Centre for Evidence-Based Medicine:
  www.cebm.net
- Clinical Governance Research and Development Unit:
  www.le.ac.uk/cgrdu
- Cochrane Collaboration Home Page:
  www.cochrane.org
- Health Information Research Unit (HIRU):
  http://hiru.mcmaster.ca
- TRIP+ database:
  www.tripdatabase.com
- Trawling the net (an introduction to free databases of interest to NHS staff):
  www.shef.ac.uk/scharr/ir/trawling.html
- ONMEDICA (information portal for GPs):
  www.onmedica.net

Further reading

- Baker M, Maskrey N, Kirk S. *Clinical Effectiveness and Primary Care*. Oxford: Radcliffe Medical Press; 1997 (out of print).
- Chambers R, Wakley G. *Making Clinical Governance Work for You*. Oxford: Radcliffe Medical Press; 2000.
- Crombie IK. *The Pocket Guide to Critical Appraisal*. London: BMJ Publishing Group; 1996.
- Dunning M *et al. Turning Evidence into Everyday Practice*. London: The King's Fund; 1998.
- Greenhalgh T. *How to Read a Paper: the basics of evidence-based medicine* (3e). Oxford: Blackwell; 2006.

- The Information Centre: Information Catalogue www.ic.nhs.uk/
- Jones R, Kinmonth AL (eds). *Critical Reading for Primary Care*. Oxford: Oxford University Press; 1995.
- Kobelt G. *Health Economics: an introduction to economic evaluation* (2e). London: Office of Health Economics; 2002.
- Lennox A, Bonser W, Robinson D, Muneer M. *A Practical Guide for Involving the Public in Health and Social Care Services*. Leicester: Leicester Promotions; 2004.
- Muir Gray JA. *Evidence-Based Healthcare* (2e). Edinburgh: Churchill Livingstone; 2001.
- Ridsdale L. *Evidence-Based General Practice: a critical reader*. London: Saunders; 1995.
- Sackett D, Strauss S, Richardson S *et al*. *Evidence-Based Medicine: how to practice and teach EBM* (2e). Edinburgh: Churchill Livingstone; 2000.
- van Zwanenberg T, Harrison J (eds). *Clinical Governance in Primary Care* (2e). Oxford: Radcliffe Medical Press; 2004.

REFERENCES

1   NHS Executive. *Promoting Clinical Effectiveness*. London: NHS Executive; 1996.

2   Hicks N. Evidence-based health care. *Bandolier* 1997; **4(5)**: 8.

3   Sackett DL, Rosenberg WM, Muir Gray JA *et al*. Evidence based medicine: what it is and what it isn't. *BMJ* 1996; **312**: 71–2.

4   Haynes RB, Sackett DL, Muir Gray JA *et al*. Transferring evidence from research into practice: 1. The role of clinical care research evidence in clinical decisions. *Evid Based Med* 1996; **1(7)**: 196–7.

5   Haynes RB, Sackett DL, Cook DJ *et al*. Transferring evidence from research into practice: 4. Overcoming barriers to application. *Evid Based Med* 1997; **2(3)**: 68–9.

6   Dunning M, Abi-Aad G, Gilbert D *et al*. *Turning Evidence into Everyday Practice*. London: King's Fund; 1997.

7   McColl A, Smith H, White P *et al*. General practitioners' perceptions of the route to evidence based medicine: a questionnaire survey. *BMJ* 1998; **316**: 361–5.

8   Samuel O. Evidence-based general practice: what is needed right now. *Audit Trends* 1997; **5**: 111–15.

9   Prescott K, Lloyd M, Douglas HR *et al*. Promoting clinically effective practice: general practitioners' awareness of sources of research evidence. *Fam Pract* 1997; **14**: 320–5.

10 Paterson C. Problem setting and problem solving: the role of evidence-based medicine. *J Roy Soc Med* 1997; **90**: 304–6.

11 Wye L, McClenahan J. *Getting Better with Evidence*. London: King's Fund; 2000.

12 Hughes J, Humphrey C, Rogers S *et al*. *Evidence into Action: changing practice in primary care*. Occasional Paper 84. London: Royal College of General Practitioners; 2002.

13 Department of Health. *Coronary Heart Disease. National Service Frameworks*. London: Department of Health; 2000.

14 National Institute for Clinical Excellence. *Compilation. Summary of Guidance issued to the NHS in England and Wales*. Issue 10. London: National Institute for Clinical Excellence; 2005. www.nice.org.uk

15 Black N. Evidence based policy: proceed with care. *BMJ* 2001; **323**: 275–9.

16 Royal College of General Practitioners. *Portfolio-based Learning in General Practice: a report of a working group on higher professional education*. Occasional Paper 63. London: RCGP; 1993.

17 Treasure W. Portfolio-based learning pilot scheme for general practitioner principals in South East Scotland. *Educ Gen Pract* 1996; **7**: 249–54.

18   Burrows P, Millard L. Personal learning in general practice. *Educ Gen Pract* 1996; **7**: 300–5.

19   Gillies A. *The Clinician's Guide to Surviving IT*. Oxford: Radcliffe Publishing; 2006.

20   *The Cochrane Library*. www.nelh.nhs.uk/cochrane.asp

21   Brenner SH, McKinin EJ. CINAHL and MEDLINE: a comparison of indexing practices. *Bull Med Lib Assoc* 1989; **77**: 366–71.

22   Okuma E. Selecting CD-ROM databases for nursing students: a comparison of MEDLINE and the Cumulative Index to Nursing and Allied Health Literature (CINAHL). *Bull Med Lib Assoc* 1994; **82**: 25–9.

23   Watson MM, Perrin R. A comparison of CINAHL and MEDLINE CD-ROM in four allied health areas. *Bull Med Lib Assoc* 1994; **82**: 214–16.

24   Kiley R. Medical databases on the Internet – part 2. *J Roy Soc Med* **90**: 679–80.

25   Kiley R. How to get medical information from the Internet. *J Roy Soc Med* 1997; **90**: 488–90.

26   Kiley R. Evidence-based medicine on the Internet. *J Roy Soc Med* 1998; **91**: 74–5.

27   *Mentor Plus* is available from www.mentorplus.com/

28   Muir Gray JA. *Evidence-based Healthcare* (2e). Edinburgh: Churchill Livingstone; 2001.

29   Carter Y, Howe A, Shaw S (eds). *Health Economics*. Master Classes in Primary Care Research No 9. London: Royal College of General Practitioners; 2005.

30   Kobelt G. *Health Economics: an introduction to economic evaluation* (2e). London: Office of Health Economics; 2002.

31   Kiley R. *The Doctor's Internet Handbook* (2e). London: Royal Society of Medicine; 2000.

32   Greenhalgh T. How to read a paper: the Medline database. *BMJ* 1997; **315**: 180–3.

33   Greenhalgh T, Taylor R. How to read a paper: papers that go beyond numbers (qualitative research). *BMJ* 1997; **315**: 740–3.

34   Hoddinott P, Pill R. A review of recently published qualitative research in general practice. More methodological questions than answers? *Fam Pract* 1997; **14**: 313–19.

35   Patton MQ. *Qualitative Evaluation and Research Methods*. London: Sage; 1990.

36   Mays N, Pope C (eds). *Qualitative Research in Health Care* (3e). London: BMJ Publishing Group; 2006.

37   Mays N, Pope C. Qualitative research in health care. Assessing quality in qualitative research. *BMJ* 2000; **320**: 50–2.

38   Murphy E, Dingwall R, Greatbatch D *et al.* Qualitative research methods in health technology assessment: a review of the literature. *Health Technol Assess* 1998; **2(16)**: 1–274.

39　Waddell G, McIntosh A, Hutchinson A *et al. Low Back Pain Evidence Review.* London: Royal College of General Practitioners; 1999.

40　Chambers R, Wakley G. *Making Clinical Governance Work for You.* Oxford: Radcliffe Medical Press; 2000.

41　Halligan A. *Clinical Governance – assuring the sacred duty of trust to patients.* Leicester: Clinical Governance Support Team; 2005.

42　Wakley G, Chambers R, Field S. *Continuing Professional Development: making it happen in Primary Care.* Oxford: Radcliffe Medical Press; 2000.

43　National Patient Safety Agency. *Seven Steps to Patient Safety. A guide for NHS staff.* London: NPSA; 2003.

44　Audit Commission. *Early Lessons in Implementing Practice Based Commissioning.* London: Audit Commission; 2006.

45　Royal College of General Practitioners. *Quality Team Development.* London: RCGP; 2000. www.rcgp.org.uk/

46　General Medical Council. *Management for Doctors.* London: General Medical Council; 2006.

47　Royal College of General Practitioners. *Access to General Practice Based Primary Care.* London: RCGP; 2000.

48　Deegan M, Hensher M and colleagues on Local Hospitals Profit Board. *Strengthening Local Services: the future of the acute hospital.* London: National Leadership Network; 2006.

49　Dunning M, Abi-Aad G, Gilbert D *et al. Experience, Evidence and Everyday Practice.* London: King's Fund; 1999.

50　Taylor M. *Unleashing the Potential. Bringing residents to the centre of regeneration.* York: Joseph Rowntree Foundation; 1995.

51　Chambers R, Boath E, Drinkwater C. *Involving Patients and the Public: how to do it better* (2e). Oxford: Radcliffe Medical Press; 2003.

52　Department of Health. *The Caldicott Committee Report on the Review of Patient-identifiable Information.* London: Department of Health; 1997.

53　Donald P. Promoting local ownership of guidelines. *Guidelines in Practice* 2000; **3**: 17.

54　Department of Health. *Standards for Better Health.* London: Department of Health; 2004.

55　Cox J, King J, Hutchinson A, McAvoy P. *Understanding Doctors' Performance.* Oxford: Radcliffe Publishing; 2006.

56　Britten N, Stevenson FA, Barry CA *et al.* Misunderstandings in prescribing decisions in general practice: qualitative study. *BMJ* 2000; **320**: 484–8.

57　Mohanna K, Chambers R. *Risk Matters in Healthcare.* Oxford: Radcliffe Medical Press; 2000. (Out of print)

58　Moore A, McQuay H. Statin safety: a perspective. *Bandolier* 2006; **13(5)**: 2–3.

59   Chambers R, Wakley G. *Clinical Audit in Primary Care. Demonstrating quality and outcomes*. Oxford: Radcliffe Publishing; 2005.

60   Lugon M, Singleton C. Chronic disease management and the implications for clinical governance. *Clinical Governance Bulletin* 2005; **6(2)**: 1–3.

61   Sheldon T, Cullum N, Dawson D *et al*. What's the evidence that NICE guidance has been implemented? Results from a national evaluation using time series analysis, audit of patients' notes, and interviews. *BMJ* 2004; **329**: 999–1004.

62   Chambers R, Wakley G, Blenkinsopp A. *Supporting Self-care in Primary Care*. Oxford: Radcliffe Publishing; 2006.

63   Healthcare Commission. *Annual Healthcheck*. London: Healthcare Commission; 2005. www.healthcarecommission.org.uk/annualhealthcheck

64   Wall D, Halligan A, Deighan M, Cullen R. Leadership, strategy and clinical governance. *Nexus Background* 2002; **4**: 1–7.

65   National Audit Office. *Achieving Improvements through Clinical Governance*. London: National Audit Office; 2003. www.nao.gov.uk/publications/nao_reports/02-03/02031055.pdf

66   James A. Making space for clinical governance. *Impact in Bandolier* 2000; **7(3)**: 5–6.

67   www.concordat.org.uk

68   Department of Health. *Research Governance Framework for Health and Social Care* (2e). London: Department of Health; 2005. Available on www.dh.gov.uk

INDEX

abbreviations, and search headings 15–16
access to services 93–4
accountability 88, 98–9
AgeLine 14
Agency for Health Care Policy and Research (AHCPR) 15
Aggressive Research Intelligence Facility (ARIF) 116
AIDSDRUGS 14
AIDSLINE 14
AIDSTRIALS 14
allied health literature, online information sources 13–14
alternative medicine, online information sources 14–15
AMED (Allied and Alternative Medicine) 14–15
annual appraisals 90, 99
annual health checks (Healthcare Commission) 103–6
applying evidence to practice 82–5
appraisals 90, 99
ARIF (Aggressive Research Intelligence Facility) 116
ASSIA plus (Applied Social Sciences Index and Abstracts) 15
*asterisk use in searches (Cochrane Library) 36
audit and evaluation 88, 89, 99, 100

Bandolier 8, 99, 115
barriers to implementing change 84–5, 106–7
Bath Information and Data Service (BIDS) 16
'benefits' 20
bias 51, 61
biological sciences, online information sources 15
British Medical Journal, online access 18
broadband access 12
browsers 12
'buddy' learning systems 10

CANCERLIT 15
Centre for Evidence Based Medicine (Oxford), website 17
Centre for Reviews and Dissemination (CRD) 116–17
change management 83–5
identifying barriers 84–5, 106–7
chemoprophylaxis 102
chronic disease registers 92
CINAHL (Cumulative Index to Nursing and Allied Health Literature) 13–14
clinical audit 6
see also audit and evaluation
clinical decision making
components 6
tools and aids 17, 99, 115
see also evidence-based healthcare
clinical effectiveness
and cost-effectiveness 20
cycle model 28
described 5
implementation principles 82–5
information sources 115–18
Clinical Evidence (NLH) 15, 115
clinical governance
components 86–8
core requirements 101
defined 86
implementation challenges 88–9
integration of components 91–102
information sources 115–18
and continuing professional development (CPD) 89–90
and risk management 89
organisation's perspectives 102–8
performance action plans 104–6
research frameworks 108–10
Clinical Governance bulletins 115
clinical questions see question formation
clinical support systems see clinical decision making
The Clinician's Guide to Surviving IT (Gillies) 12
co-mentors 10

Cochrane Central Register of Controlled
Trials (CENTRAL) 13
Cochrane Database of Systematic Reviews
(CDSR) 29, 30–1
Cochrane Library 12–13, 30–1, 48–9
search examples 36, 38–9, 41–2
techniques 43–4, 48–9
cohort studies 54
communication issues, patient–doctor
misunderstandings 99
complementary medicine, online
information sources 14–15
conclusions, critical analysis 61
confidence intervals 51–2
confidentiality 88, 96
conflicts of interest 61
confounders 52
continuing professional development
(CPD) 89–90
controlled trials 52
controls, defined 52
coronary heart disease 104–5
cost minimisation 20
cost-benefit analysis (CBA) 20, 52
cost-effectiveness analysis (CEA) 20–2, 52
cost-minimisation analysis (CMA) 52
cost-utility analysis (CUA) 20, 53
CPD (continuing professional
development) 89–90
critical appraisal 59–62
bias concerns 61
defined 51
evidence 'hierarchies' 32–3
interpretation aids 99
methodology issues 59–60
validity concerns 61
worked examples 62–81
of published papers 59–72
of qualitative research 73–5
of reports 59–72
of reviews 75–81
cross-sectional surveys 54
Cumulative Index to Nursing and Allied
Health Literature (CINAHL) 13–14

data requirements 7
standards 92–3
Database of Abstracts of Reviews of Effects
(DARE) 13, 29
demographic data 7

design of studies, critical analysis 58, 59–60,
61
Dialog 50
disease registers 92
disease risk factors 96
$ sign (Medline) 39–40
'double blind' trials 56
Drug & Therapeutics Bulletin (DTB) 115

economic evaluations, types 20
EDINA BIOSIS 15
effectiveness, defined 53
efficacy, defined 53
efficiency, defined 22
electronic journals 17–18
Elsevier 13
EMBASE (Excerpta Medica database) 13
EMIS (Egton Medical Information Systems
Ltd) 17
evidence appraisal *see* critical appraisal
evidence 'hierarchies' 32–3
evidence-based healthcare
attitudes towards 8–9
criticisms 9
culture changes in practice 97–8, 102–8
described 5–6
effectiveness 6–7
information sources 115–16
methods and processes 6
organisation's perspectives 102–8
outcomes 7
training needs 9
and clinical governance 88, 102–8
and research governance
frameworks 108–10
Evidence-Based Medicine 115–16

file transfer protocol (ftp) 12
'fit to practice' standards 98
focusing searches 38

'grey' literature 40

Hawthorne effect 53
health gains 88, 96
Health on the Net (HON) 16
health promotion 88, 99
Health Technology Assessment Database
(HTA) 13
Healthcare Commission 103

Healthcare Concordant 108
healthcare information 7
    data standards 92–3
healthcare variability 88–9
hierarchy of evidence 32–3
hospital trusts
    approaches to clinical governance 102–6
    goals and targets 104
    performance action plans 104–6
    threats to implementation 106–8
*HSTAT (Health Services/Technology
    Assessment Text)* 116
hypertext transfer protocol (http) 12

immunisations 102
incidence, defined 53
information searches
    advice and training 29
    formulating questions 19–20, 22–6
    grading the evidence 32–3
    key strategies 28–9
    techniques 29–32, 43–5
information sources
    CINAHL 13–14
    Cochrane Library 12–13, 30–1, 43–4,
        48–9
    EMBASE (Excerpta Medica database) 13
    Medline 12, 31–2, 44–5, 49–50
    other sites 16–17
    subject specific bibliographic
        databases 14–16
intention to treat analysis 53
Internet
    search advice 12–18
    set-up in healthcare settings 11–12
    use by patients 7
    see also information searches; information
        sources
Internet Service Providers (ISPs) 12

journals online *see* electronic journals;
    information sources

key words 29–31
    with Cochrane Library searches 30–1
    with Medline searches 31
King's Fund
    on identifying barriers to change 85
    on implementation of evidence-based
        practice 9

learning cultures 87, 91
    applying R & D 92
librarians 29, 40
lifelong learning 89–90
literature searches
    advice and training 29
    basic techniques 29–32, 43–5
    deciding aims and questions 19–20,
        22–6
    grading the evidence 32–3
    key strategies 28–9
    knowing when to stop 42
    using key words 29–31
    worked examples 33–45

MedHunt 16
medical abbreviations, and search
        terms 15–16
Medical Matrix 16
Medline 12, 31–2
    search examples 33–5, 37–8, 39–41
    techniques 32, 44–5, 49–50
Mentor Plus 17
mentors 10
MeReC Bulletin 116
MeSH (Medical Subject Heading) terms
        31
    worked examples 33–5
meta-analysis, defined 54
methodology issues, critical appraisals
        59–60
Microsoft Internet Explorer 12
misunderstandings 99
modifiable risk factors 96

National Institute for Health and Clinical
        Excellence (NICE) 117
National Library for Health (NLH) 13
National Research Register (NRR) 16
National Service Frameworks 105
Navigator 12
Netting the Evidence 116
NHS Centre for Reviews and Dissemination
        (CRD), information availability 16
NHS Economic Evaluation Database
        (NHSEED) 13
NLM Gateway 17
numbers needed to treat (NNT) 53
nursing literature, online information
        sources 13–14

observational studies 54
odds ratio (OR) 54
OldMedline 17
omissions in research 62
opportunity costs 20

'*p*' values 55–6
PACE initiative (King's Fund) *see* Promoting
    Action on Clinical Effectiveness (PACE)
patient empowerment 7
patient involvement 7, 87, 94–6
patient population data 7
   standards 92–3
patient–doctor misunderstandings 99
performance evaluations 88
   and accountability 98–9
   and clinical governance 89
   data needs 7
   Healthcare Commission's annual health
     checks 103–6
   see also underperformance
placebos 54
portfolio-based learning 9–10
power calculations 59
   defined 54–5
PreMedline 17
prevalence 55
preventative treatments 102
primary care organisations
   approaches to clinical governance 102–6
   goals and targets 104
   performance action plans 104–6
   threats to implementation 106–8
probability 55–6
Promoting Action on Clinical Effectiveness
   (PACE) 6–7, 85
Proquest 18
psychology, online information sources 15
PsycINFO® 15
public consultation 94–6
public health, online information sources 15
publication bias 56
PubMed 12, 16–17

qualitative research, critical appraisals 73–5
'quality' 22
Quality and Outcomes Frameworks 105
Quality Practice Awards 90
Quality Team Development 90
quality-adjusted life-years (QUALYs) 20, 53

question formation
   general guidance 19–20
   identifying issues 47
   framing words 47–8
   choosing and using key words 29–30, 48
   worked examples 22–6
questionnaires 60

randomised controlled trials 56
   and bias 61
reading research papers 58–9
ReFeR (Dept of Health Research Findings
   Register) 16
relative risks 56–7, 99
reliability 57
research governance frameworks 108–10
   see also evidence-based healthcare
research terminology 51–8
resource management 93–4
response rates 60–1
results, critical appraisals 60
retrospective recall 59
revalidation 98
reviews, critical appraisals 75–81
risk management 88, 89, 101–2
   see also health gains
risk ratios 56–7
root word searches 36, 39
Royal College of General Practitioners,
   Fellowship awards 90

sample sizes 54–5
saving searches 50
search strategies 28–9
search techniques 29–32, 43–5
self-assessment questionnaires 2–4
sensitivity analysis 57
sensitivity of tests 57
service management standards 93–4
significance 55–6
skill-mix models 93
social sciences, online information
    sources 15
software
   Mentor Plus 17
   Web Mentor Library 17
specificity of tests, defined 57
sponsorship concerns 61
Standards for Better Health (DoH 2004) 103
star ratings 103

statistically significant, defined
    57
stopping searches 42
SUMSearch 15
systematic reviews 29, 30–1
    defined 57

team working 87, 94
training in evidence-based practice,
    perceived needs 9
TRIP+ database 17

underperformance 88–9
    identification and remedies 99

validity 58
    critical appraisal 61

Web Mentor Library 17
website information sources 117
Wiley publishers 13
workplace standards 93–4
World Wide Web (www) 12